PERGAMON INTERNATIONAL LIBRARY
of Science, Technology, Engineering and Social Studies

*The 1000-volume original paperback library in aid of education,
industrial training and the enjoyment of leisure*

Publisher: Robert Maxwell, M.C.

TREATING CHILDHOOD AND ADOLESCENT OBESITY

PSYCHOLOGY PRACTITIONER GUIDEBOOKS

EDITORS

Arnold P. Goldstein, Syracuse University
Leonard Krasner, Stanford University and SUNY at Stony Brook
Sol L. Garfield, Washington University

TREATING CHILDHOOD AND ADOLESCENT OBESITY

DANIEL S. KIRSCHENBAUM
Northwestern University Medical School

WILLIAM G. JOHNSON
University of Mississippi Medical Center

PETER M. STALONAS, JR.
University of Rochester

PERGAMON PRESS
New York   Oxford
Beijing   Frankfurt   São Paulo   Sydney   Tokyo   Toronto

Pergamon Press Offices:

U.S.A.   Pergamon Press, Maxwell House, Fairview Park, Elmsford, New York 10523, U.S.A.

U.K.   Pergamon Press, Headington Hill Hall, Oxford OX3 0BW, England

PEOPLE'S REPUBLIC OF CHINA   Pergamon Press, Qianmen Hotel, Beijing, People's Republic of China

FEDERAL REPUBLIC OF GERMANY   Pergamon Press, Hammerweg 6, D-6242 Kronberg, Federal Republic of Germany

BRAZIL   Pergamon Editora, Rua Eça de Queiros, 346, CEP 04011, São Paulo, Brazil

AUSTRALIA   Pergamon Press (Aust.) Pty., P.O. Box 544, Potts Point, NSW 2011, Australia

JAPAN   Pergamon Press, 8th Floor, Matsuoka Central Building, 1-7-1 Nishishinjuku, Shinjuku-ku, Tokyo 160, Japan

CANADA   Pergamon Press Canada, Suite 104, 150 Consumers Road, Willowdale, Ontario M2J 1P9, Canada

---

First printing 1987

Library of Congress Cataloging in Publication Data

Kirschenbaum, Daniel S., 1950-
    Treating childhood and adolescent obesity.

    (Psychology practitioner guidebooks)
    Includes index.
    1. Obesity in children. 2. Obesity in children--
Treatment. 3. Behavior therapy for children.
I. Johnson, William G., 1939- . II. Stalonas,
Peter M. III. Title. IV. Series.
RJ399.C6K52 1986   618.92'3'98   86-25436
ISBN 0-08-032414-2
ISBN 0-08-032413-4 (soft)

Printed in Great Britain by Hazell Watson & Viney Limited, Aylesbury, Bucks

To the memory of our cherished friend and colleague, Peter M. Stalonas, Jr.

Contents

Preface

Behavior therapists have been pursuing the treatment of obesity with great dedication since the late 1960s. After Richard Stuart documented the successful treatment of eight obese women in 1967, it seemed that all we had to do was continue to focus on modifying eating habits and the result would be many healthier and happier formerly overweight adults. Unfortunately, adult obesity showed itself to be far more refractory than originally anticipated. Dozens of controlled studies revealed that a wide array of biological and behavioral barriers occur that prevent overweight adults from successfully and permanently losing weight.

The authors were among the many behavior therapists who began treating and studying adult obesity and related self-regulatory problems in the late 1960s and 1970s. Mirroring the rest of the field, we, too, became discouraged with the relatively modest long-term success rates obtained in our treatment outcome studies. We began working with overweight children because we thought that early intervention might lead to better outcomes. After all, if one works with children and their parents, it might be possible to redirect behavioral patterns before they become entrenched and to modify the social context in which efforts at behavior change take place. The extant literature on the treatment of obese children has generally supported this view: by working rather intensively with overweight children and their parents for an extended period of time (6 months at least), long-term success can be achieved in many, perhaps most, cases.

The purpose of this guidebook is to help other clinicians use the accumulated research and clinical knowledge about the treatment of childhood and adolescent obesity. This is a relatively young field (only a decade or so old), but the time is right to share the knowledge about the elements of successful programs. This book attempts to accomplish the goal of sharing that information in several ways. First, an introductory chapter reviews the literature, with an emphasis on the elements of treatment programs that seem to lead to the best outcomes. Six elements were discovered that appear especially useful: active parental involvement, increased exercise, prolonged and intense treatment, modification of eating style, use of behavioral contracts, and certain therapist characteristics. The operational meaning of these elements and other key issues (e.g., definition and measurement of obesity in children and adolescents) are discussed in that first chapter. Second, we provide explicit guidelines for both experienced and novice clinicians for how to conduct up to 100 sessions for groups of overweight children and their parents. Third, we include copies of the extensive handouts we provide to both children and their parents during the treatment program. The handouts contain a variety of forms needed for working on habit change, as well as basic information on such topics as nutrition, generating and maintaining commitment, coping with stress without using eating as a response, and goal setting, planning, and problem solving. Finally, the appendix consists of program application forms and guidelines for conducting assessment interviews with both parents and children.

All of the materials in this book have been used extensively in several clinical sites: treatment programs and research studies conducted at the University of Rochester, University of Wisconsin–Madison, University of Mississippi Medical Center, and Northwestern University School of Medicine. As we discuss in chapter 1, the results obtained with the approach suggested in this book have been very promising. We hope that the provision of this very explicit account of how to conduct an effective weight–control program for children and adolescents will encourage more research in this area (now that the independent variable, i.e., nature of the treatment, can be identified very publicly and explicitly) as well as help clinicians in their work with this important population.

When writing this book, we realized that some clinicians and researchers might like to have copies of the client handouts made available to them. There are more than 100 pages of handouts and forms that we describe or refer to in this book. Readers who would like full-sized copies of all of the handouts (with 3-holes punched in them for easy insertion into a looseleaf book) may write for more information to Dan Kirschenbaum, PhD, Northwestern University Medical School, Department of Psychiatry and Behavioral Sciences, 320 East Huron Street, Chicago, IL 60611.

Chapter 1
Elements of Success in the Treatment of Childhood and Adolescent Obesity

SCOPE OF THE PROBLEM

Obesity among children and adolescents is clearly a serious health problem. Longitudinal studies show that higher levels of risk factors for cardiovascular disease in children correlate significantly with childhood obesity and with higher levels of such factors in adulthood. For example, in the Muscatine study of more than 4,000 Iowa children (Lauer, Connor, Leaverton, Reiter, & Clark, 1975), elevated weight and skinfold measures of fat were associated with high levels of coronary risk factors (elevated blood pressure and lipoprotein levels). Unfortunately, overweight children and adolescents are more likely to maintain their overweight status as adults, with its associated risk factors, than are their peers of normal weight (Brook, 1972; Zinner, Levy, & Kass, 1971). For example, Abraham and Nordsieck (1960) followed up 50 overweight boys and found that 86% became obese adults (approximately 15% of adult males are obese). Eighty percent of the obese girls followed up by these researchers became obese adults, versus 18% obesity in their normal-weight control group. Stunkard and Burt (1967) concluded from data such as Abraham and Nordsieck's that the odds *against* a normal-weight adulthood for those who do not reduce during adolescence are 28:1.

It seems clear that people who hope that an obese child will "grow out of it" are awaiting an unlikely event. Approximately 5% to 20% of the children and adolescents in this country meet one of several possible criteria that define them as obese (LeBow, 1984). Because they will not grow out of their obesity, these children, as well as their parents, must consider more aggressive approaches if they wish to decrease or eliminate the many problems associated with lifelong obesity. It should be emphasized that much more than physical health is at stake in this regard. The psychosocial consequences of obesity are severe and begin

1

very early in life. Obese children can expect to be rejected by their peers more than any other handicapped type of person (LeBow, 1984), possibly develop low self-esteem (Felker, 1968), develop very unfavorable views of their bodies (Mendelson & White, 1985), and experience a myriad of discriminations and rejections as adults (LeBow, 1984).

The purpose of this chapter is to examine what should be done to help obese children and adolescents lose weight based on current knowledge of the efficacy of various approaches to treating this notoriously refractory problem. The definitions and causes of childhood and adolescent obesity will be reviewed briefly before considering how to treat it. In the examination of treatments, emphasis will be placed on identifying seemingly active elements of successful treatments. The final section of this chapter will integrate this material by describing the elements and approaches that seem warranted in an idealized treatment for childhood and adolescent obesity.

DEFINITIONS AND CAUSES OF CHILDHOOD AND ADOLESCENT OBESITY

Definitions

In a variety of epidemiological studies, reported rates of childhood obesity have varied from 2% to 40% for the United States (LeBow, 1984). Much of this variance is probably due to the varying criteria used to determine obesity status. These range from arbitrary judgments of the size of "obese" skinfolds (measured by skin calipers, most often applied to the triceps) to percentile cutoffs for skinfold measures (e.g., the group with the skinfolds that place them in the top 10% of a sample), to weights considered with respect to norms for a particular age, sex, and height cohort. There is no veridical means of assessing obesity in youngsters, nor is there one commonly accepted practice. Certainly all assessments of obesity in children must take into account the fact that they grow at very significant rates. This means that use of various weight/height indexes (see Edwards, 1978; Kirschenbaum, 1986) is recommended, because these indexes incorporate normatively based growth rates in their calculations. Generally, a criterion such as "having a weight index (normed for age, sex, and height) above the 90th percentile" is an adequate means of defining childhood obesity. Percentage of overweight could be derived quite easily from weight/height index data (Kirschenbaum, 1986). A similar cutoff could be based on tables derived for measures of skinfold fatness (e.g., Seltzer & Mayer, 1965).

Whichever measurement system is used by the clinician or the researcher, it is important to emphasize that obese children who are left untreated tend to follow the adage "and the fat get fatter." This has been established in several treatment-outcome studies that included control groups (e.g., Brownell & Kaye, 1982). For example, Kirschenbaum, Harris, and Tomarken (1984) found that, over a 6-month period, untreated controls (9 to 13 year olds) gained a statistically and clinically significant 4% in overweight (from 42.4% to 46.4%). Therefore, significant reduction in percentage of overweight resulting from treatment could be clinically significant and significant relative to controls in many cases.

Causes

Before discussing how to treat childhood and adolescent obesity, it would be helpful to understand the nature of the problem we propose to treat. It is clear that many millions of children, adolescents, and adults gain excess weight and then fail in their struggles to lose it. This occurs despite formidable personal and social pressures to maintain low weight (Polivy, Garner, & Garfinkel, 1985). Why does obesity develop, and what makes it so resistant to change?

Research on the development and maintenance of obesity has made it increasingly clear that this is a complex, multidetermined problem. Genetic, biological, behavioral, familial, cultural, and economic factors interact in complex ways to affect the development and maintenance of this disorder. Selective breeding experiments and twin studies have shown strong genetic contributions (Foch & McClearn, 1980). Studies of metabolic adaptations to weight reduction (e.g., Donahoe, Lin, Kirschenbaum, & Keesey, 1984) and of adipose cells (Sjostrom, 1980) make it clear that there are substantial biological barriers working to maintain or increase weight in the obese.

A fact sometimes used to support the biological view is that children whose parents are obese are much more likely to be obese than children whose parents are lean (Garn & Clark, 1976). On the other hand, considerable evidence shows that less biologically-oriented factors contribute to the problem. For example, there are significant correlations between the weights of spouses (Garn & Clark, 1976), between the weights of pet owners and their dogs (Mason, 1970), and between measures of obesity of foster parents and their children (Garn, Cole, & Bailey, 1977). Furthermore, obese children typically show a "high density" eating style (Kirschenbaum & Tomarken, 1982), which one could argue is a behavioral contributor to obesity. This eating style includes excessive eating, with more gulping and less chewing seen in obese children than in their leaner peers. Obese children also appear less active than their leaner counterparts, at least in some studies (Brownell & Stunkard, 1980).

Apparently, many complex variables interact to determine which child will become fat and which will be lean. However, the biology of obesity indicates that a positive energy balance must exist for obesity to occur. That is, for obesity to develop, the amount of energy consumed must be greater than the amount of energy expended. The child can become obese by eating a great deal, by being very sedentary, or by a combination of the two. Or the child might have a body that efficiently captures energy from food and stores it. If one has a very efficient body in this regard, then intake can be quite normal, but a surplus of energy (calories) occurs anyway, resulting in the buildup of excess fat.

The problem faced by those who treat obesity is how to get the body to a state of negative energy balance (energy intake — energy expenditure = a negative number) and keep it there long enough to use up the excess fuel that is stored in adipocytes. Regardless of the mechanisms by which the obesity developed, this problem is a substantial one. The body seems to resist, in both subtle and obvious ways, efforts to create and sustain a negative energy balance (see Donahoe et al., 1984; Wooley, Wooley, & Dyrenforth, 1979). As we will describe later, the active elements of successful treatments for childhood and adolescent obesity include a multifaceted and intense assault on biological, behavioral, and other fronts to counter the powerful forces that operate to maintain or increase obesity in young people. The complex causes of obesity, compounded substantially by the formidable biological barriers operating against weight reduction, seem to demand this kind of intensive, sustained, multifocused treatment.

ELEMENTS OF SUCCESS

General Approach:
Behavioral versus Dietary versus ?

There have been no comprehensive long-term outcome studies comparing the effects of various approaches to the treatment of childhood obesity. *Comprehensive*, in this case, refers to those that include adequate controls for such nonspecific effects as expectancies, therapeutic style, credibility of treatment, and attention directed at target behaviors both during and subsequent to treatment sessions (cf. Kirschenbaum, Stalonas, Zastowny, & Tomarken, 1985). On the other hand, reviews of the extant literature tend to favor behavioral approaches (e.g., Brownell & Stunkard, 1980; Coates & Thoreson, 1978), as do the very encouraging outcomes obtained in some recent studies (e.g., Epstein, Wing, Koeske, & Valoski, 1984; Epstein, Wing, Woodall, Penner, Kress, & Koeske, 1985).

The study that has come closest to a comprehensive comparative outcome study (Epstein et al., 1985) deserves a closer look. Nineteen 5 to 8-year-old girls were randomly assigned to one of two intensive treatments: a behavioral or a comparison treatment. Both groups participated in a 5-week camp involving meetings for the children twice a week (all morning long) combined with weekly meetings in the evening during which parents and children were seen separately. In both groups, attendance contracts were operational (payback of deposit money contingent upon attendance), and both groups received a great deal of attention from therapists and extensive materials about health, nutrition, and exercise (including specialized diet and exercise materials, prompts, and monitoring information). The behavioral group also participated in more explicit, extensive parent training (including contracting) and received more self-monitoring instructions and materials. Thus, the behavioral treatment included not only behavioral principles and techniques but also training in child-management skills, increased attention to target behaviors outside of therapy, and perhaps, the benefit of more favorable expectancies on the part of the behaviorally oriented therapists who conducted the study and the parents who signed up for the program (which was well-known in the community for its behavioral focus). Each of these nonspecific ingredients might well have played an active role in treatment, thereby differentially affecting outcomes relative to the comparison condition (cf. Israel, Stolmaker, & Andrian, 1985; Kirschenbaum et al., 1985; Kirschenbaum & Tomarken, 1982).

Despite these issues, it should be emphasized that the authors took great pains to provide the groups with equal amounts of attention from the therapists on a number of additional dimensions (education, measurement opportunities, etc.). It is therefore important to view the outcomes they obtained as supportive of either behavioral approaches per se or of behavioral approaches that include the nonspecific elements just discussed. The magnitude of change observed was -26.3% overweight for the behavioral group, which was 2.4 times the -11.2% change observed in the comparison group. Also, the children in the treatment (behavioral) group lost, on the average, enough weight to make them no longer obese at the 1-year point (actually, 5 of the 8 children in this group became nonobese by the 1-year point). These are clinically significant outcomes, albeit with small sample sizes.

At this juncture in the history of research on treating obesity in young people, we cannot advocate unqualified acceptance of a behavioral approach, with its attendant assumptions and methods. It is true that the best outcomes in controlled trials obtained to date have been associated with behavioral treatments (the work of Epstein and his associates). Nonetheless, we do not as yet know the primary active elements that accounted for those favorable results. Did the children lose weight because, as we behaviorists might hope, they learned important self-management principles (cf. Cohen, Gelfand, Dodd, Jensen, & Turner, 1980) or because they used principles of learning to modify their problematic eating habits? Or were the behavioral treatments effective because they included active, competent leaders employing a highly credible, segmented system that promoted cooperative parent-child interactions (see Kirschenbaum et al., 1984; Kirschenbaum et al., 1985). The latter could well be crucial ingredients, but they are not conceptually linked to a behavioral approach.

The "horse race" issue (behavioral versus other approaches) must await further study at this point. For now, however, we can look to the literature for potentially active elements of treatment in an ecumenical manner with regard to theoretical orientation. Let us see what seems to be working first and then decide how best to conceptualize it. The six elements of treatment that appear most important and that will be examined next are (a) active parental involvement; (b) increased exercise; (c) prolonged and intense treatment; (d) modification of eating style; (e) use of behavioral contracts; and (f) certain therapist characteristics.

Active Parental Involvement

Families that experience frequent conflicts tend to have less adequate dietary habits than families that do not report excessive strife (Kinter, Boss, & Johnson, 1981). Conflictual families are also more likely to have children with anorexia and bulimia (Humphrey, in press.) Eating plays a central role in family life, and it is not surprising that trouble in families is associated with eating problems. This analysis also applies to the treatment of childhood and adolescent obesity. Families who reported chaotic home environments at pretreatment were more likely to drop out of treatment, in one study, than were less chaotic families (Kirschenbaum et al., 1985). Relatedly, the training of parents in child management skills, which can reduce family conflict, facilitated parent and child weight reduction, relative to weight-reduction training alone (Israel et al., 1985).

It is becoming clear that families with generalized problems and conflicts have a difficult time helping their obese children lose weight. These conflicted families need either focused training in child management or more elaborated family therapy in order to change the obesity status of their children (see Israel et al., 1985; Kirschenbaum et al., 1984). Relatively healthy families, however, also have great difficulty helping obese children and adolescents lose weight. The physiological basis of the problem is one of many factors that account for this difficulty. Fortunately, several studies have yielded useful information on how to build social support that promotes weight control in families with obese children and adolescents (e.g., Brownell, Kelman, & Stunkard, 1983; Coates, Killen, & Slinkard, 1982).

A high degree of parental involvement generally improves outcomes in parent–child weight-loss programs (Brownell et al., 1983; Coates et al., 1982; Epstein, Wing, Koeske, Andrasik, & Ossip, 1981; Kirschenbaum et al., 1984). However, these improvements can be rather small at 1-year follow-ups (e.g., Coates et al., 1982; Israel et al., 1985; Israel, Stolmaker, Sharp, Silverman, & Simon, 1984). On the other hand, parents show greater support for the weight-control effort when they are closely involved in treatment, and this can result in increased parent and child cooperation and effort, with decreased attrition (e.g., Kingsley & Shapiro, 1977; Kirschenbaum et al., 1984). Therefore, it is advisable to have parents closely involved with the treatment of their obese children. This could involve working with groups of 2 to 4 parents and their children. Or it could mean conducting separate groups for parents along with parallel child groups (Brownell et al., 1983; Cohen et al., 1980). The parent groups do not necessarily have to emphasize the parents' own weight-control problems (Epstein et al., 1981; Israel et al., 1984). They can focus on how parents can be effective helpers for their children. They could also focus on the parents' own use of the program's techniques that help them modify eating and exercise habits in order to lose weight.

Increased Exercise

It is becoming very clear that weight-control interventions must focus on increasing exercise in addition to the traditional goal of changing eating patterns. The evidence suggests that increasing exercise can prevent a metabolic adaptation to dieting that interferes with sustained weight loss (Donahoe et al., 1984). Exercise might also decrease appetite. Epstein, Masek, and Marshall (1978), for example, found that including a 10-minute exercise period before lunch reduced the caloric intake of six obese children just as effectively as nutritional education. These effects, and others, probably contribute to success in weight reduction (e.g., Dahlkoetter, Callahan, & Linton, 1979; Stalonas, Johnson, & Christ, 1978; see also Thompson, Jarvie, Lahey, & Cureton, 1982). These converging bits of evidence have led to the inclusion of exercise in almost all current behavioral treatment programs for obesity. In contrast, during the 1960s and 1970s, only 10% of the treatment-outcome studies on obesity included explicit emphasis on increased exercise (Wing & Jeffery, 1979).

The problem with trying to increase the frequency and intensity of exercising in relatively sedentary people is that they usually do not maintain their increased activity patterns for more than a few months (Dishman, 1986). A variety of interventions might help prevent this type of self-regulatory failure (Kirschenbaum, 1986). For example, people tend to maintain exercise regimens better if they enjoy the type of exercise, if the exercise is convenient for them to use, and if the exercise includes other people (Dishman, 1986). These points could be incorporated when encouraging children to increase their exercising.

Epstein and his colleagues conducted two studies designed to test various ways of increasing exercise in obese children (Epstein, Wing, Koeske, Ossip, & Beck, 1982; Epstein, Wing, Koeske, & Valoski, 1985). In both studies, children who engaged in "life-style exercising" lost more weight at the final follow-up assessment (17 and 24 months post-treatment, respectively) than children in "programmed exercise" groups. The life-style exercisers earned points that corresponded to calories expended for various activities that had not been engaged in prior to the study (e.g., walking to and from school). The programmed group used similar numbers of points as their targets and accumulated them by following a preplanned exercise routine (e.g., swimming every day after school).

In some ways it is difficult to tell if the life-style exercise approach tested by Epstein and his colleagues was superior to the programmed approach. The programmed approach invoked an inflexible (proximal and specific) plan. That type of plan generally does not facilitate self-regulation as well as a more distal and moderately specific plan (Kirschenbaum, 1985). Perhaps programmed exercising could have produced very good results if it had been encapsulated in a plan that used the principles of effective planning more closely. This might have involved getting the overweight children to establish goals such as "participate in three extra gym classes per week" or "play soccer 3 times a week." These are not everyday or life-style exercise regimens, but for many children they might have desirable features, such as enjoyment and involvement with others. Also, the latter plans are flexible (more appropriate in terms of proximity and specificity; that is, they do not require exercising every day or on specific days or times). Therefore, these plans could have produced some of the favorable results expected from more intensive workouts (e.g., increased musculature; maintenance of more helpful metabolic rates).

Perhaps the best advice to therapists is to encourage the use of moderately specific and relatively distal (weekly, not daily) planning to increase exercising in both programmed and life-style approaches (see Martin et al., 1984). Children could plan to participate in team sports, join teams or leagues of various kinds, and increase and monitor their life-style exercising. It would probably help a good deal if parents modeled high levels of exercise and participated with their children in physical activities as much as possible.

Prolonged and Intense Treatment

People vary a great deal in their response to treatments for obesity. This fact qualifies all of the empirically based recommendations we can offer. Therefore the suggestion that longer term and more intensive interventions generally produce at least somewhat more favorable outcomes includes no guarantees as to how this approach will affect each client. It does seem reasonably clear that, if all other factors are equal (e.g., treatment modality, emphasis on exercise), it is desirable to meet with obese clients *at least once a week for 8 to 12 months*, longer if needed. This recommendation is supported by comparing the results obtained in relatively long-term studies with studies that were more time-limited (see Craighead, Stunkard, & O'Brien, 1981; Wadden, Stunkard, & Brownell, 1983). For example, Kirschenbaum et al. (1984) noted that the weight losses achieved by children in their 9-week program (−6.1% change in percentage of overweight) was comparable to other behavioral programs of similar duration and superior to controls, who typically gained weight over that period of time. In contrast, behavioral programs that last for 6 or 8 months often produce 2 to 3 times greater weight reduction (e.g., Epstein et al., 1981).

Extended and relatively intensive programs probably facilitate weight change because they help clients maintain their self-monitoring of food intake, exercise expenditure, and weight and promote continued use of other self-regulatory strategies (Coates & Thoresen, 1981; Kirschenbaum, 1986; Sandifer & Buchanan, 1983; Stalonas & Kirschenbaum, 1985). Perri and his associates (Perri, McAdoo, Spevak, & Newlin, 1984; Perri, Shapiro, Ludwig, Twentyman, & McAdoo, 1984), for example, recently showed that sustained therapist contact (weekly) can facilitate maintenance of key behavioral strategies and improve weight loss, relative to various comparison conditions. If weight reduction is viewed as a complex behavioral and biological struggle, it makes perfect sense that long-term treatment is necessary. Weekly contact probably should be sustained for several months after goal-weights are achieved, to help promote generalization of behavior changes. We cannot point to an empirical justification for the latter recommendation in large part, because, unfortunately, goal weights have rarely been achieved in controlled clinical trials.

Modification of Eating Style

Obese children tend to exhibit a high density eating style more than their leaner peers (Kirschenbaum & Tomarken, 1982). *High density eating* refers to eating rapidly, taking big spoonfuls or big mouthfuls of food, and gulping food by chewing relatively little for the amount of food consumed. This eating style can increase the body's propensity to store excess nutrients as fat (Collier, Hirsch, & Hamlin, 1972). Also, high density eating prevents elongation of the chain of behaviors involved in the eating process. Elongation of the eating chain, or *chaining*, is the kind of deliberate, slow eating style that people in behavioral weight-control programs usually attempt to achieve. Use of chaining and related strategies that enhance awareness of the eating process probably increases the likelihood of successful weight control (Coates & Thoresen, 1981; Sandifer & Buchanan, 1983; Stalonas & Kirschenbaum, 1985).

The evidence just cited suggests that focusing on the eating styles of obese children could be a helpful component of treatment programs. Probably the key method of helping children and adolescents modify their eating styles is the promotion of self-monitoring of food intake. Research on self-regulatory failure clearly indicates that when the process of systematically obtaining information about a target behavior begins to break down or stop, people tend to discontinue effective self-regulation. This principle probably holds for weight regulation by young people. For example, Flanery and Kirschenbaum (1986) conducted a retrospective study of children who had participated in a weight-loss program 1 to $1^1/2$ years prior to the assessment. Of the 11 habit-change strategies assessed, only sustained use of self-monitoring (according to both child and parent reports) was clearly associated with long-term success. Therefore, the treatment of obese children and adolescents probably should include emphasis on the changing of eating styles and on sustained self-monitoring of eating behavior.

Use of Behavioral Contracts

There have been more studies of the effects of behavioral contracting on weight control than on any other target behavior (Kirschenbaum & Flanery, 1983). The evidence generally encourages continued use of behavioral contracts and accelerated study of their active elements.

A behavioral contract is "an explicit agreement specifying expectations, plans, and/or contingencies for the behavior(s) to be changed" (Kirschenbaum &

Flanery, 1983, p. 224). The four central elements of behavioral contracting are (a) form of the contract (e.g., written versus verbal, negotiated, individualized, public); (b) contract participants; (c) target behaviors (e.g., process versus outcome goals); and (d) consequences. To date, we know relatively little about which of these elements are active ingredients in behavior change (see also Kirschenbaum & Flanery, 1984). Nonetheless, the evidence shows that contracting facilitates weight reduction relative to minimal (e.g., self-monitoring only) or no treatment and that focusing on habit-change goals rather than on weight-loss goals can prove beneficial (Kirschenbaum & Flanery, 1983). It also seems desirable to have clients write out their own contracts each week (with a consultation with the therapist) and to include in those contracts weekly goals that are challenging yet achievable and plans that are moderate in specificity (Kirschenbaum & Flanery, 1984). For example, clients could include in their contracts "to self-monitor every day; to list 80% of the calories; to jog 3 times this week; to enter my weight on my weight-loss graph once; to remove ice cream and other dessert foods from my house." These goals and plans do *not* include weight-loss outcomes (e.g., "to lose 2 lbs") nor are they too specific (e.g., "to jog Tuesday, Thursday, and Saturday mornings"). The consequences of achieving contracted goals could be set at a modest sum (e.g., return $2 a week of a deposit for success and $2 for attendance), because amount of the consequences usually does not determine efficacy (Kirschenbaum & Flanery, 1983). In work with obese children, consequences should probably include many positive social events and responses. For example, consequences could include trips to the zoo, walks in the park, ice skating, or special privileges at home. It might help to have the child complete the Children's Reinforcement Survey (Phillips, Fischer, & Singh, 1977) to generate many good ideas for consequences that could prove motivating.

Certain Therapist Characteristics

Obese clients have rated behavior therapists superior to nonbehavior therapists in competence and potency in several studies (e.g., Harmatz & Lapuc, 1968; Wollersheim, 1970). Some of these differential ratings are probably due to the number and types of behavioral techniques suggested, the credibility of the jargon used to describe them, and, perhaps, the increased amount of attention paid to the specific efforts made by each client. Whether or not these therapist characteristics make a substantial difference in long-term outcomes remains unknown.

The fact that some therapist characteristics *do* make a difference in the treatment of obesity is consistent with studies of therapist characteristics in general (see Goldstein & Myers, 1985) and with the experience of those who have trained many novice therapists (e.g., Dubbert & Wilson, 1983; Kirschenbaum et al., 1985). Two studies also documented the potency of therapist effects on long-term weight-loss outcomes (Beneke & Paulsen, 1979; Kirschenbaum et al., 1985). In the latter study, a therapist pair that clients rated as more "democratic" (less "authoritarian") after the second group meeting obtained superior outcomes 2 years later compared to those obtained by a therapist pair viewed as less democratic (more authoritarian). Perhaps the more successful pair of therapists helped the clients understand that they were continuously making choices about their eating and exercising, whereas the less successful therapists provided more direct advice about what clients should do. The former emphasis, on *protracted choice*, has facilitated other self-regulated behavior changes (Kirschenbaum, Tomarken, & Ordman, 1982), including weight reduction (Loro, Fisher, & Levenkron, 1979). This enhanced focus on self-directedness could prove especially important when clients must learn to maintain and otherwise generalize changes initiated in therapy (Kirschenbaum, 1985). This analysis must be viewed with caution, however, prior to replications and experimental manipulations of such therapeutic styles.

These data and observations indicate that the clinical context in which obese children and adolescents are treated probably deserves attention. Providing a set of materials with some superficial explanations is unlikely to lead to substantial changes in obesity. Therapists probably need to develop very effective clinical skills, perhaps including emphasis on the choices clients make when trying to change eating and exercising patterns. It might also make sense to screen clients for interpersonal abilities prior to forming groups (e.g., 5 to 6 people per group). This idea could improve the quality of group interactions and facilitate adequate amounts of attention for each participant.

SUMMARY: ELEMENTS TO INCLUDE IN AN IDEALIZED TREATMENT PROGRAM

The previous sections document the fact that we cannot base treatment plans for childhood and adolescent obesity on data alone. However, six ingredients are apparently worth including, based on existing research and educated speculation: active parental involvement, a focus on increasing exercise, prolonged and intense treatment, attempts to modify problematic (e.g., high density) eating styles, behavioral contracting, and high-level clinical skills of therapists (in particular, emphasis on choices by clients).

These elements combine to yield a program of intervention in which potential group members (children and parents) are screened for compatibility with the approach. Then, children and their parents are seen together in groups of 2 or 3 parent–child dyads, or children and parents are seen in their own groups, with 5 or 6 peers per group. The groups are conducted by a skillful clinician (or a closely supervised professional trainee), and they meet weekly for 6 to 18 months. Group members are encouraged to commit to weekly attendance well beyond the point at which they reach goal weights (e.g., 2 or 3 months of weekly maintenance meetings). Each week, each participant writes a new behavioral contract. The contracts focus on process goals (e.g., habit changes, not weight loss) and include explicit contingencies to encourage sustained attendance and effort. One key focus in each contract is on increasing exercise. Explicit weekly exercise goals are just as important as goals to change high density eating styles.

The idealized treatment presented thus far does not include a specific set of topics or a theoretical orientation. Perhaps it is not vitally important to do more than use the six elements discussed earlier. However, methods of changing eating and exercising styles are incorporated most comprehensively in behavioral approaches. Behavioral approaches also differentially emphasize the idea that *change is possible, desirable, and achievable.* Such an emphasis encourages people to work harder at personal development (e.g., Farina, Fisher, Getter, & Fischer, 1978). Finally, explicit treatment manuals are available to help guide the clinician and to specify independent variables for the researcher (for adults: Johnson & Stalonas, 1981). Therefore, unless alternative approaches become more explicit and convincing, behavioral approaches to the treatment of childhood and adolescent obesity seem useful at this time. Behavioral approaches are, by no means, the panaceas they were once believed to be. However, they do provide the best available medium for including the elements that seem most important when working with overweight children, adolescents, and their parents.

The remainder of this book contains all that a skilled clinician needs to conduct a weight-control program for children and adolescents. It includes instruction on how to cover the content of 10 lessons to be used by parents and children. Handouts for clients are also provided. They include all of the necessary tables and forms to be used by clients to self-monitor, plan, and use other techniques. Finally, the appendix contains the forms and instructions needed to screen potential clients.

Chapter 2
Session 1.
Generating the Commitment
to Lose Weight

INTRODUCTION

Leader's Goals: To help clients begin to feel comfortable in the group; to make being in the group a positive, enjoyable experience.

Activities: Discussion, warm-up exercise.

First, review the leader's goals with the group—the importance of getting to know each other, so that you begin feeling comfortable together. Next, conduct a warm-up exercise of some sort. For example, group leaders could introduce themselves by giving their names plus some activity each of them likes to do (e.g., dancing, volleyball). The person to the right of the group leader is asked to repeat the leader's name and associated activity and then give his or her name and an activity to be associated with him or her. The third person's task is to give the group leader's name and activity plus the second person's name and activity and then give his or her name and an activity. This process continues all around the group until it reaches the group leader again, who then attempts to repeat everyone's name and activity. Alternatively, group members could pair off and talk with each other for several minutes. Their goal should be presented as getting enough information to allow each one to introduce his or her partner to the group. After 10 minutes, reconvene the whole group and ask them to provide introductions for their partners.

COMMITMENT: THE BALANCE
SHEET PROCEDURE

Leader's Goal: To help clients begin to make active, logical choices about losing weight.

Activities: Completion and discussion of decision balance sheets.

13

Step 1. Ask Open-ended Questions

Ask your clients to talk about why they want to lose weight. For example, you might ask, "What are the best and the worst things for you about trying to lose weight?"

Step 2. Introduce the Balance Sheet

Explain to your clients, "Talking about the 'whys' of weight reduction is important. But, to really make an informed, highly committed choice, you need to consider all possible pros and cons concerning this difficult decision. Listing all the pros and cons on a 'balance sheet' can help people do that." Before asking your clients to complete a balance sheet, have them think of specific weight-loss goals they wish to reach. These could be simply a number of pounds, a change in percentage of overweight, or a given number of pounds over a specific number of weeks or months.

Step 3. Have Clients Complete
an Initial Balance Sheet

Have your clients complete a decision balance sheet such as the one in Figure 2.1. They need to list the goal under consideration from Step 2 and then all the items relevant to the eight categories shown on the blank balance sheet. This can be done with a therapist or by the clients alone and then reviewed with other clients and the therapist. This is a brainstorming technique. Therefore, make sure your clients consider *all* ideas as "good" or "ok" and place them on their balance sheets.

FIGURE 2.1. Decision Balance Sheet — Type I

Name: _____	Date: _____
Goal: _____	
Tangible Gains/Losses to Self	
Positive Anticipations	*Negative Anticipations*
1.	1.
2.	2.
3.	3.
4.	4.
5.	5.
6.	6.
7.	7.
8.	8.
9.	9.
10.	10.

FIGURE 2.1. Decision Balance Sheet — Type I (continued)

Tangible Gains/Losses to Others

Positive Anticipations	Negative Anticipations
1.	1.
2.	2.
3.	3.
4.	4.
5.	5.
6.	6.
7.	7.
8.	8.
9.	9.
10.	10.

Self Approval/Disapproval

Positive Anticipations	Negative Anticipations
1.	1.
2.	2.
3.	3.
4.	4.
5.	5.
6.	6.
7.	7.
8.	8.
9.	9.
10.	10.

Social Approval/Disapproval

Positive Anticipations	Negative Anticipations
1.	1.
2.	2.
3.	3.
4.	4.
5.	5.
6.	6.
7.	7.
8.	8.
9.	9.
10.	10.

Comments:

Step 4. Refine the Balance Sheet

Review Figures 2.1 and 2.2 with your adult clients and Figures 2.3 and 2.4 with your young clients. Use ideas in these examples to generate additional items for your clients' balance sheets. See if any of the items in Figures 2.2 and 2.4 seem relevant to your clients. Incorporate the relevant ideas on your clients' balance sheets. For example, see if your adult client did *not* include from Figure 2.2 item 10 under "Tangible Gains/Losses to Self: Positive Anticipations." This item, "Spend less money on fad diets," should be discussed with your client. For example, "Is this relevant to you?" "How much money did you spend in the past year or two on specialized diets?" If the item is germane, ask your client to write a version of this (and any other relevant items from Figure 2.2 or 2.4) on her or his balance sheet.

FIGURE 2.2. Example of an Adult's Weight-Loss Balance Sheet

Name: Jan L.   **Date:** 2/21/85

Goal: To lose 50 lbs. in 1 year

Tangible Gains/Losses to Self

Positive Anticipations	*Negative Anticipations*
1. Improve ability to walk around — shop, hike.	1. Takes lots of time to count calories, food.
2. Improve tennis game.	2. Costs money for group sessions, exercise classes.
3. Increase contact with others.	3. Exercising could cause injuries.
4. Improve health over long run (live longer!).	4. Takes time to keep records and do exercises.
5. Increase job opportunities.	5. Costs money for new clothes.
6. Be able to buy more stylish clothes.	6.
7. Be able to borrow others' clothes.	7.
8. Go to the beach more.	8.
9. Get presents other than stationery (like clothes!).	9.
10. Spend less money on fad diets and specialized diet foods.	10.

Tangible Gains/Losses to Others

Positive Anticipations	*Negative Anticipations*
1. Increased socializing (helping others, being a friend).	1. I might burden others with need for support.
2. More energy for family.	2. Others in family will have to do more cooking.
3. More willing to do active things with family.	3. I'll be busier — with exercising and group sessions — so have less time for others.

FIGURE 2.2. Example of an Adult's Weight-Loss Balance Sheet (continued)

4. More expertise available for family in nutrition, exercise, self-control.	4. There will be fewer "treats" available in the house.
5. More expertise available for friends.	5. There will be less money available for others.
6. Might live longer, so I can help my family longer.	6.
7. More healthful foods and life-style modeled by me for family.	7.
8.	8.
9.	9.
10.	10.

Self Approval/Disapproval

Positive Anticipations	Negative Anticipations
1. Feel proud.	1. Feel too "obsessed."
2. Feel more self-confident.	2. Feel restricted.
3. Feel sense of mastery.	3. Become less joyful and spontaneous.
4. Feel in control of my body.	4. Feel as though I have bought into cultural pressures to be thin.
5. Understand my body and myself better.	5. Feel too much like a "health nut."
6.	6.
7.	7.
8.	8.
9.	9.
10.	10.

Social Approval/Disapproval

Positive Anticipations	Negative Anticipations
1. Friends will congratulate me.	1. Friends could think my dieting is weird.
2. Relatives will recognize my strengths.	2. Friends and relatives might not want me to change.
3. People will see me as a person first, not just as a "fat person."	3. Some people might become jealous of me.
4. Kids won't laugh at me anymore.	4. When I refuse to eat certain things at dinners and parties, hosts will feel hurt.
5. Spouse will find me more attractive.	5. Family might not like my decreased willingness to bake or go out for desserts.

FIGURE 2.2. Example of an Adult's Weight-Loss Balance Sheet (continued)

6. Others will find me more attractive.	6.
7. Friends will like my less depressed, happier disposition.	7.
8.	8.
9.	9.
10.	10.

Comments:

Step 5. Evaluate the Items

Have clients rate the importance of each item. Use a scale such as, 1 (not too important) to 3 (very important). Define importance as something valued very highly due to impact, consequences, or personal meaning. Discuss examples of very important and not-too-important things. During the group session, have each client read his or her key items on both positive and negative sides.

FIGURE 2.3. Decision Balance Sheet — Type II

Name: _____	Date: _____
Goal: _____	
Good Things About Trying to Reach the Goal and About Reaching the Goal	Bad Things About Trying to Reach the Goal and About Reaching the Goal
1.	1.
2.	2.
3.	3.
4.	4.
5.	5.
6.	6.
7.	7.
8.	8.
9.	9.
10.	10.
11.	11.
12.	12.
13.	13.
14.	14.
15.	15.

FIGURE 2.4. Example of a Youngster's Weight-Loss Balance Sheet

Name: Pat P.   **Date:** 2/21/85

Goal: To lose 20 lbs in 1 year

Good Things About Trying to Reach the Goal and About Reaching the Goal	Bad Things About Trying to Reach the Goal and About Reaching the Goal
1. Become better able to play sports.	1. Takes a lot of time to lose weight.
2. Become a faster runner.	2. Might feel worse if I fail.
3. Feel better about myself.	3. Others might laugh at me for dieting.
4. Like the way I look in clothes.	4. Others might get mad at me for not eating like they do.
5. Be better able to find clothes I like.	5. Might change my view of myself.
6. Find that other people will like me more.	6. Will be hard to keep myself from eating foods that I like.
7. Undergo less teasing from others.	7.
8. Feel proud of myself.	8.
9. Feel stronger.	9.
10. See parents become proud.	10.
11. Spend less money on food.	11.
12. Save money for other things.	12.
13. Understand myself better.	13.

Step 6. Encourage Clients to Make the Decision

Have clients total all of the positive and all of the negative ratings. If the positive score is clearly higher than the negative score, the decision to pursue the goal makes a lot of sense. Commitment to it should be enhanced. Clients should keep their balance sheets with their self-monitoring forms or post them near their weight graphs. They should be reviewed regularly, and therapists should retain a copy of each client's sheets. When motivation tends to fade later in the weight-loss effort, the balance sheets can be reviewed again, redone, or used to create a list of self-statements to be read several times a day (perhaps pair them to drinking coffee, water, or diet soda or to eating meals).

If the positive items do not clearly outweigh the negative items, several issues emerge. Perhaps the goal needs to be redone (e.g., target less weight loss over a longer period of time). Or, most important, perhaps the negatives are simply too potent for the individual. If subsequent discussion with the group or therapist does not change this view, the client probably should not attempt to lose weight. The client might need help adjusting to the social pressures of being overweight. Or the client simply is not appropriate for treatment and should be encouraged to feel good about thoroughly considering the available options. The decision *not* to lose weight should be considered viable and reasonable by the therapist in most cases, due to the great difficulty of the weight-loss process and the relatively minor health risks associated with certain forms of obesity (e.g., 20% overweight constitutes relatively few physical health risks for most people). In any event, *the person who cannot make a very clear commitment to lose weight is virtually guaranteed to fail at any such attempt.* This is as true for children as it is for adults. Therapists might wish to keep this concept in focus, especially when working with parents and children. Children, however, might become better able to make a commitment to weight loss after very carefully redoing a balance sheet within the context of a good relationship with a therapist. This probably would not be necessary for most obese adults who are seeking help. The latter group usually has little difficulty making a strong commitment to weight loss.

ELEMENTS OF SUCCESS
IN WEIGHT CONTROL

Leader's Goals: To introduce clients to the philosophy and principles to be used in this program; to help clients understand the approach and develop a commitment to using it actively and effectively.

Activities: Discussion of causes of weight problem, group rank ordering of four key causes; discussion of implications.

1. *MY BODY—not MYSELF.* Ask participants what factors cause their *current* weight problems. Have the group discuss this in pairs. Structure the discussions by having the pairs rank in order of importance several potential causes of weight problems. Consider suggesting the following potential causes to be included in the rankings:
   (a) *abnormal eating habits:* eating the wrong foods, eating too fast, eating too late at night, snacking too often, not exercising enough.
   (b) *family/culture:* living in a society that emphasizes high-calorie fast foods, learning to eat in a problematic fashion in the family (e.g.,not eating breakfast), being in a culture or subculture that tends to eat high-calorie low-protein foods.
   (c) *genetics/physiology:* having a low metabolic rate, having inherited a tendency to gain weight easily from parents and grandparents.
   (d) *personality:* tending to eat in response to stress and other emotions, being neurotic, having problems with feelings about oneself, being depressed or anxious.

   For *children*, this needs simplification. The four categories could be as follows:
   (a) *food and exercise:* the kind of food I eat, how much I exercise.
   (b) *family and friends:* how my family and friends eat and exercise, their style of eating, and how important they consider eating and exercising to be.
   (c) *emotions:* eating because of feeling upset.
   (d) *biology:* something being wrong with my body so that I seem to gain weight faster and easier than others who seem to eat and exercise just like I do.

After the pairs discuss these factors, get the whole group together to share the outcome of the discussions. Put the four potential causes on the blackboard. Figure out their average rankings, from least to most important as perceived causes.

When discussing these rankings make the following points:

- The number 1 ranking should be *physiology/genetics*, which plays a *very important* role in causing and maintaining problems with excess weight. Use Figure 2.5 to help make this point.
- Family/culture can play a role (e.g., there is three times more obesity in lower socioeconomic groups in this country, but three times more people on diets in higher socioeconomic status groups; children adopted by obese parents are more likely to be obese than those adopted by lean parents).
- Personality can affect eating and weight. But being overweight is not a sign of personal weakness or neurosis. Excess weight is a *physiological problem* or challenge. Overcoming it requires the kind of behavioral skills needed to change one's biology — one's body. Losing weight is not the same, for most people, as trying to change one's personality via psychotherapy. It requires changing the body in a manner very similar to the changes worked on by highly dedicated athletes. You need to train yourself and your body to overcome its natural tendencies. All good athletes do exactly the same thing. For example, the great football player, Walter Payton, did not have legs that "wanted" to grow to look like tree trunks; he had to *make* those changes occur through a long-term commitment and hard work. (Show Figure 2.5 to emphasize the point that problematic physiology *can be overcome*.)
- The results of difficult physiology and certain family/cultural factors (and, to a much lesser extent, personality factors) are eating and exercising patterns that usually are *not abnormal*. For example, overweight adults usually do not eat much, if any, more than people of normal weight. The physiology of obesity makes it much easier for overweight people to maintain their excess weight or increase their weight compared with people who have never had weight problems. So, in order to lose weight, overweight people must develop an eating and exercising pattern that is abnormally stringent. These changes can be achieved, but they are changes that are supernormal (more difficult, more restrictive, etc.) than the eating patterns used by most non-obese people. Again, emphasize that *losing weight is like training for athletic competition*.

2. *Implications for this Program*
   (a) The "blame" for weight problems goes largely to one's biology, not to one's self. You are *ok* (at least!); your body simply needs to be trained, just like an athlete's body needs to be trained.
   (b) We focus on difficult and permanent changes in life-style (eating and exercising).

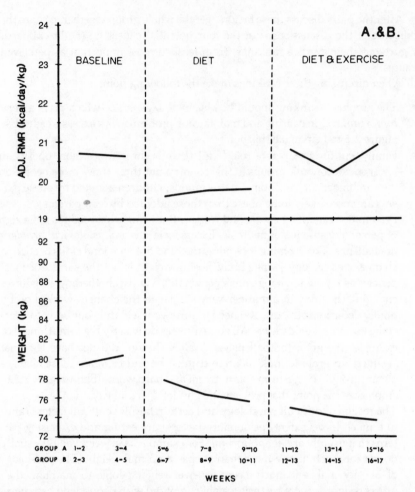

FIGURE 2.5. Adjusted Resting Metabolic Rate (RMR/kg) and Weight Across Treatment Phases. (Each point is the mean of four measures averaged over the 8 subjects completing all three phases.) The RMR data show that when people reduce their caloric intake by dieting, their metabolic rates often decline dramatically. However, if they exercise regularly (as in the Diet & Exercise phase above), their metabolic rates can return to normal. A slowed down metabolic rate can make it very difficult to lose weight. Thus, the body resists losing weight when people go on diets, but this biological resistance can be overcome by exercising. From "Metabolic Consequences of Dieting and Exercise in the Treatment of Obesity" by C.P. Donahoe, Jr., D.H. Lin, D.S. Kirschenbaum, and R.E. Keesey, 1984, *Journal of Consulting and Clinical Psychology, 52,* p. 830. Copyright 1984 by American Psychological Association.

(c) The "training" in this program involves:
   (1) learning and mastering certain self-management skills to improve your effectiveness as a "body trainer;"

(2) learning to solve problems effectively;

(3) giving and receiving support, encouragement, and constructive ideas;

(4) using the group to provide a little external pressure.

HOMEWORK ASSIGNMENT

Leader's Goal: To get clients thinking about and working on relevant tasks during the week.

Activities: Provision of information and a handout, discussion of the week's tasks.

1. Distribute Handout 1 and discuss its key points as a summary of issues raised during the session.

2. Explicitly go over the material in Handout 1 on definitions of overweight. Have the participants determine their weight goals.

3. Make the following assignments for this week (also listed on the last page of Handout 1):

   (a) encourage parents and children to read and discuss Handout 1. Ask them to set aside some specific time to do this (e.g., after dinner midweek).

   (b) have parents and children cut out 1 to 3 "weight loss" ads from newspapers or magazines and bring them in next week.

   (c) ask participants to complete their decision balance sheets and bring them back next week.

   (d) have clients begin their own weight graphs. The Y-axis should include a range of only 10 to 20 lbs. The X-axis should be labeled "dates." Have clients enter one weight per week and write in the date as they enter the weight. Do not have them pre-plan when to weigh themselves. Just enter a date and weight about once per week.

BEHAVIORAL CONTRACTS

Leader's Goal: To improve compliance and accelerate progress.

Activities: Formation and discussion of first contracts.

1. *Introduction.* Explain that it is necessary to set specific goals each week in order to make effective changes in eating and exercising patterns. Everyone in this program will need to establish new goals each week to help her or him reach those goals. This is like homework; however, the participants in the group are responsible for deciding their own homework assignments. There is no teacher here who will make those decisions.

2. *Format.* Each participant should write out specific goals each week, using carbon paper or pressure-sensitive, noncarbon copy paper. The group leader

should keep a copy, and the clients should be asked to post their copies in a closet or some other place in their homes where they will see them every day.

3. *Procedure.* Toward the end of each session, allocate several minutes for writing and discussing behavioral contracts. In this first session, have clients review Figure 2.6 as an example. Note on the example that the client signed the contract and dated it. Also note that each element of the contract is numbered. Inform the clients that this contract, like all others in this program, was written by the client, and the goals established in it were decided upon by the client, with the therapist and other group members serving as consultants and helpers.

FIGURE 2.6. Sample Behavioral Contract

March 6, 1985

For this week, I will:

1. Self-monitor food (amounts) and calories at least 6 out of 7 days.
2. Self-monitor exercise (calories burned) for the week (enter a new point on my weekly exercise graph).
3. Use stimulus control by eating only in the kitchen (or in restaurants) for at least 4 days.
4. Jog at least twice for at least 30 minutes.
5. Enter 1 or 2 new weights on my weight graph.

Pat Smith

4. *Guidelines for Writing Contracts.* The following points can help improve the efficacy of contracting:
   (a) Emphasize that the *choices* of which goals to focus upon are being made by the client.
   (b) Encourage clients to select *achievable* but somewhat challenging goals. These should be goals they believe they can achieve but that are still somewhat difficult.
   (c) Make sure the goals are *process*, not *outcome*, goals. That is, the goals should include behavior changes people can make that should effect the outcome goal of losing weight. Goals to increase exercise by a certain amount, to self-monitor for a certain number of days, and to practice other behavioral strategies (e.g., taking time-outs when eating; using stimulus control concepts), are good examples of process goals. Outcome goals could include these: to lose a certain number of pounds, to fit

into a certain pair of pants, and to get a compliment from someone on one's new appearance.

(d) Establish *consequences* for attendance and for achieving goals. Tables 2.1 and 2.2 include lists of potential reinforcers for parents and children, respectively. These can be provided to parents and children to help them generate ideas for consequences to use in their contracts. For parents and children, you could return deposit money contingent on attendance and successful achievement of goals. You could use $1 to $3 returned per week for attending the session and a similar amount for achieving contracted goals. A related approach of particular use with parents is to have the parents provide you with a number of small checks (e.g., $1 to $3 each) written to a disfavored political cause or a charity they do not particularly like. These checks could be mailed out contingent on attendance and goal attainment. For children, a token system could be used so that they can accumulate tokens to be exchanged for desired purchases each week or saved for bigger items over a longer period of time.

5. *The First Contract.* As in Figure 2.6, the first contract could specify such items as reviewing Lesson 1, posting the decision balance sheet, and updating the balance sheet at least once during the week.

Table 2.1. Potential Rewards for Adults

Being in the country	Going to lectures or hearing speakers
Wearing expensive or formal clothes	Driving skillfully
Making contributions to religious, charitable, or other groups	Breathing clean air
Talking about sports	Thinking up or arranging songs or music
Meeting someone new of the same sex	Taking tests when well prepared
Going to a rock concert	Boating (canoeing, kayaking, motorboating, sailing, etc.)
Playing baseball or softball	Planning trips or vacations
Pleasing my parents	Buying things for myself
Restoring antiques, refinishing furniture, etc.	Being at the beach
Doing artwork (painting, sculpture, drawing, moviemaking, etc.)	Watching TV
Rock climbing or mountaineering	Talking to myself
Camping	Working in politics
Reading the scriptures or other sacred works	Working on machines (cars, bikes, motorcycles, tractors, etc.)

Table 2.1. Potential Rewards for Adults (continued)

Playing golf	Thinking about something good in the future
Taking part in military activities	Playing cards
Rearranging or redecorating my room or house	Completing a difficult task
Going to a sports event	Laughing
Reading a how-to book or article	Solving a problem, puzzle, crossword, etc.
Going to the races (horse, car, boat, etc.)	Being at weddings, baptisms, confirmations, etc.
Reading stories, novels, poems, or plays	Having lunch with friends or associates
Playing tennis	Going to a bar, tavern, club, etc.
Taking a shower	Taking a nap
Driving long distances	Being with friends
Woodworking, carpentry	Canning, freezing, making preserves, etc.
Solving a personal problem	Writing stories, novels, plays, or poetry
Being in a city	Being with animals
Taking a bath	Riding in an airplane
Exploring (hiking away from known routes, spelunking, etc.)	Singing to myself
Having a frank and open conversation	Making food or crafts to sell or give away
Singing in a group	Playing pool or billiards
Thinking about myself or my problems	Being with my grandchildren
Working on my job	Playing chess or checkers
Going to a party	Pursuing a craft (pottery, jewelry, leather, beads, weaving, etc.)
Speaking a foreign language	Going to church functions (socials, classes, bazaars, etc.)
Going to service, civic, or social club meetings	Putting on makeup, fixing my hair, etc.
Going to a business meeting or a convention	Designing or drafting
Being in a sporty or expensive car	Visiting people who are sick, shut in, or in trouble
Playing a musical instrument	Cheering, rooting

Table 2.1. Potential Rewards for Adults (continued)

Making snacks	Bowling
Snow skiing	Being popular at a gathering
Combing or brushing my hair	Watching wild animals
Acting	Having an original idea
Reading essays or technical, academic, or professional literature	Gardening, landscaping, or doing yard work
Wearing new clothes	Getting massages or back rubs
Dancing	Receiving letters, cards, or notes
Sitting in the sun	Watching the sky, clouds, or a storm
Riding a motorcycle	Going on outings (to the park, on a picnic, to a barbecue, etc.)
Just sitting and thinking	Playing basketball
Buying something for my family	Drinking socially
Seeing good things happen to my family or friends	Practicing photography
Going to a fair, carnival, circus, zoo, or amusement park	Giving a speech or a lecture
Talking about philosophy or religion	Reading maps
Gambling	Gathering natural objects (wild foods, rocks, driftwood, etc.)
Planning or organizing something	Working on my finances
Having a drink by myself	Making a major purchase or investment (car, appliance, house, stocks, etc.)
Dating, courting, etc.	Listening to the sounds of nature
Having a lively talk	Helping someone
Listening to the radio	Racing in a car, motorcycle, boat, etc.
Having friends come to visit	Hearing jokes
Playing in a sporting competition	Winning a bet
Introducing people who I think would like each other	Talking about my children or grandchildren
Giving gifts	Meeting someone new
Talking about my health	Going to school or government meetings, court sessions, etc.

Table 2.1. Potential Rewards for Adults (continued)

Seeing beautiful scenery	Being in a fraternity or a sorority
Improving my health (having my teeth fixed, getting new glasses, changing my diet, etc.)	Being with my parents
Being downtown	Horseback riding
Wrestling or boxing	Protesting social, political, or environmental conditions
Hunting or shooting	Talking on the telephone
Playing in a musical group	Having daydreams
Hiking	Kicking leaves, sand, pebbles, etc.
Playing lawn sports (badminton, croquet, shuffleboard, horseshoes, etc.)	Going to a museum or an exhibit
Doing a job well	Writing papers, essays, articles, reports, memos, etc.
Having spare time	Going to school reunions, alumni meetings, etc.
Fishing	Seeing famous people
Loaning something	Going to the movies
Being noticed as sexually attractive	Kissing
Pleasing employers, teachers, etc.	Being alone
Cooking meals	Budgeting my time
Counseling someone	Being praised by people I admire
Going to a health club, sauna, etc.	Outwitting a "superior"
Learning to do something new	Having someone criticize me
Complimenting or praising someone	Doing a project in my own way
Being told I am needed	Doing odd jobs around the house
Being at a family reunion or get-together	Thinking about people I like
Washing my hair	Giving a party or get-together
Coaching someone	Thinking about other people's problems
Going to a restaurant	Playing board games (Monopoly, Scrabble, etc.)
Seeing or smelling a flower or plant	Sleeping soundly at night

Table 2.1. Potential Rewards for Adults (continued)

Being invited out	Doing heavy outdoor work (cutting or chopping wood, clearing land, farming, etc.)
Receiving honors (civic, military, etc.)	Reading the newspaper
Having someone agree with me	Using cologne, perfume, or after-shave
Reminiscing, talking about old times	Snowmobiling or dune-buggy riding
Getting up early in the morning	Being in a body-awareness, sensitivity, encounter, therapy or rap group
Having peace and quiet	Dreaming at night
Doing experiments or other scientific work	Playing ping-pong
Visiting friends	Brushing my teeth
Writing a diary	Swimming
Being counseled	Playing football
Saying prayers	Running, jogging, or doing gymnastic, fitness, or field exercises
Giving massages or backrubs	Walking barefoot
Hitchhiking	Playing frisbee or catch
Meditating or doing yoga	Doing housework or laundry; cleaning things
Seeing a fight	Being with my roommate
Doing favors for people	Listening to music
Talking with people on the job or in class	Arguing
Being relaxed	Knitting, crocheting, embroidering, or doing fancy needlework
Being asked for my help or advice	Petting, necking
Talking about sex	Amusing people
Going to a barber or a beautician	Talking about politics or public affairs
Having house guests	Asking for help or advice
Reading magazines	Being with someone I love
Sleeping late	Talking about my hobby or special interest
Starting a new project	Watching attractive women or men
Having sexual relations	Being stubborn

Table 2.1. Potential Rewards for Adults (continued)

Having other sexual satisfactions	Playing in the sand, a stream, the grass, etc.
Going to the library	Talking about other people
Playing soccer, rugby, hockey, lacrosse, etc.	Being with my husband or wife
Preparing a new or a special food	Going on field trips, nature walks, etc.
Birdwatching	Expressing my love to someone
Watching people	Shopping
Building or watching a fire	Smoking tobacco
Winning an argument	Caring for houseplants
Selling or trading something	Having coffee, tea, or a coke with friends
Finishing a project or a task	Taking a walk
Repairing things	Collecting things
Sewing	Playing handball, paddleball, squash, etc.
Bicycling	Working with others as a team
Playing party games	Remembering a departed friend or loved one; visiting a cemetery
Writing letters, cards, or notes	Doing things with children
Being complimented or told I have done well	Beachcombing
Being told I am loved	Attending a concert, an opera, or a ballet
Staying up late	Playing with pets
Having family members or friends do something that makes me proud of them	Going to a play
Being with my children	Looking at the stars or the moon
Going to auctions, garage sales, etc.	Being coached
Doing volunteer work; working on community service projects	Thinking about an interesting question
Receiving money	Receiving money
Hearing a good sermon	Defending or protecting someone; stopping fraud or abuse
Winning a competition	Picking up a hitchhiker
Talking about my job or school	Making a new friend

Table 2.1. Potential Rewards for Adults (continued)

Borrowing something	Reading cartoons, comic strips, or comic books
Seeing old friends	Traveling with a group
Using my strength	Teaching someone
Going to office parties or departmental get-togethers	Traveling

Note: Adapted from "Pleasant Events Schedule Form III-S" in "The Pleasant Events Schedule: Studies on Reliability, Validity and Scale Intercorrelations," by D.J. MacPhillamy and P.M. Lewinsohn, 1982, *Journal of Consulting and Clinical Psychology, 50,* pp. 363–371. Copyright 1982 by D.J. MacPhillamy. Adapted by permission.

Table 2.2. Potential Rewards for Children

Playing with racing cars	Playing with electric trains
Playing with matchbox cars	Bicycling
Playing with dolls	Watching TV—favorite programs
Watching movies—Westerns, horror, comedy	Listening to favorite records
Seeing a play or a puppet show	Playing football—with other kids, with a parent or parents
Swimming	Bowling
Skating	Skiing
Playing basketball	Riding horses
Playing tennis	Hiking
Playing chess	Playing checkers
Fishing	Playing baseball
Playing ping-pong	Shooting pool
Playing a musical instrument	Singing
Dancing	Drawing
Building models	Working with tools
Working with clay	Riding in the car
Going to work with a parent	Visiting relatives
Making a visit to the seashore	Going on a family picnic
Vacationing with the whole family	Vacationing with parents only
Going on an airplane ride	Taking a family bicycle ride
Visiting a friend	Visiting a new city
Visiting a museum	Taking a trip to a sports event
Taking a walk in the woods	Going to the store
Playing with friends	Hunting for frogs, snakes, etc.
Being hugged or kissed	Being praised by father, mother, teacher, or friend
Having a friend sleep over	Belonging to Scouts or other clubs
Taking music lessons	Learning a new language

Table 2.2. Potential Rewards for Children (continued)

Setting the table	Doing school work: reading, spelling, science, social studies, gym, math
Baking cookies	Making the bed
Working in the garden	Repairing or building
Picking flowers	Going on errands
Putting on makeup	Getting new clothes
Dressing up in mother's clothes	Dressing up in a costume
Going to a beauty parlor	Getting a haircut
Staying up past bedtime	Reading books for pleasure
Having free time	Earning money
Having a party	Having a pet
Getting an allowance	Going to a party

HANDOUT 1: SHOULD
YOU LOSE WEIGHT?

Thin Crazy

During the past 10 years or so Americans have become thin crazy. Everywhere you look there are advertisements for new diets and new exercise programs and there are very thin women modeling the latest fashions. Thin is definitely "in."

Some people think that this "thin craziness" is actually a good thing. After all, they argue, thinness means healthiness. Many people think that those who are thin eat sensibly, exercise regularly, and encourage others to do the same. Indeed, the scientific evidence clearly shows that good amounts of exercising and proper nutrition are beneficial to our health.

Unfortunately, thin craziness has gone too far. A recent study showed that the average Miss America candidate and the average Playboy Playmate have become much taller and thinner over the last 20 years. These models of the "ideal woman" are now so thin that, if the trend continued for 100 years on its current course, the average ideal woman would be so thin that she would barely be alive! This emphasis on thinness has probably caused a tremendous increase in two serious eating disorders among young women. Many more girls and young women today are starving themselves to dangerously low weights, and others are locked into a cycle of binge eating and purging (vomiting or using laxatives after eating). These eating problems, called *anorexia nervosa* (starving oneself) and *bulimia* (binge eating and purging), produce many physical and emotional problems. Certainly we do not want people to use this program to help themselves become too thin, or to help themselves adopt a new and crazy standard of thinness.

Facts about Fatness

This program is intended for young people and adults whose weight is too high for their health and well-being. Being overweight can produce unpleasant effects on your health, your ability to get along with others, and your feelings about yourself.

Effects of Obesity on Physical Health. Most people think that being overweight is quite dangerous and that greater health risks are associated with greater amounts of excess weight. Indeed, being overweight does make it more likely that you will develop certain medical problems, including diabetes, hypertension, hyperlipidemia, kidney stones, and musculoskeletal problems. On the other hand, being only a few pounds overweight might not substantially increase the risk of developing heart disease or of dying. For example, a 10-year follow-up study of more than 12,000 men in seven countries found no relationship between weight and risk of coronary heart disease in most weight categories. The only exception to this was that being very overweight and being extremely thin were associated with the development of serious health problems.

Even if being overweight does not increase the risk of certain medical problems; compared with thin people, that does not mean that losing weight might not be beneficial. When overweight people lose weight, they improve their chances of *not* developing diabetes and hypertension. Weight loss is associated with decreased cholesterol in the blood and decreased symptoms of diabetes and high blood pressure. These changes can improve your chances of living a longer and healthier life. Many overweight and obese people could increase their long-term health by losing weight.

Effects of Obesity on Relationships with Others. Many people believe obese people are generally lazy, stupid, and weak. This stereotype results in children rejecting other children who are overweight. Adults also react to obese individuals in a prejudicial fashion. For example, in one study, obese people had more difficulty renting an apartment than similar people who were not overweight. In other experiments, overweight people had difficulty gaining admission to colleges and, in a recent study, in being treated appropriately by rehabilitation counselors. These effects are particularly strong for girls and women. It seems that overweight people are treated as second-class people by many others.

How Overweight Are You? Definition. The terms *obesity* and *overweight* have no absolute definitions. Experts and researchers choose as "ideal weights" those that are associated with the greatest long-term health, based on large-scale studies. However, people vary in the size of their bones and the development of their muscles. So, a very trim and muscular 5′ 5″ gymnast could weigh as much as a 5′ 5″ businessman who is obviously overweight. This occurs because muscles weigh much more than fat for the same amount of tissue. Similarly, people with large wrists, backs, and ribcages (large *bone structures* or *builds*) can be at healthy weights that are higher than healthy weights for people of the same height who have smaller bone structures.

These variations in bodily build mean that you must know whether your build is large or small to use tables of desirable or ideal weights to judge the degree to which you are overweight. In the most widely used of these tables for adults, the 1983 Metropolitan Height and Weight Tables, the ideal weight for a 5′ 2″ man (with no clothes) is 131 lbs, with a range of from 123 lbs to 145 lbs considered appropriate, depending on the size of the man's *frame* (bone structure, build). Men can calculate their ideal weights from this table by using the 5′ 3″ medium-frame midpoint of 133 as a starting point. Add 3 lbs for every inch of height above 5′ 3″. This gives the midpoint without clothes for men of medium builds. However, ideal weights can be 10 to 15 lbs less for small builds and 10 to 15 lbs more for large builds. For women, use the 4′ 10″ midpoint of 112 lbs (no clothes) and add 2 or 3 lbs for every inch above that height. Again, desirable weights will vary by as much as 10 to 15 lbs lower or higher than the midpoint, depending on bone structure. For boys and girls between 8 and 16 years old, use Figure 2.7.

FIGURE 2.7. A Measure of Overweight for Boys and Girls

1. What is your height? (in inches)
2. What is your weight? (in pounds)
3. Divide your weight by your height. This gives you your "weight–height ratio."
4. This table shows the weight–height ratios for boys and girls who are 8 to 18 years old. If your ratio is *higher* than the 95% number for your age and sex, you are probably overweight. Remember, if you have a large build, you might have a high ratio but still be at a good weight. However, if you have a very small build, you can be overweight even if your ratio is at the 50% level.

	Boys		Girls	
Age	50th percentile*	95th percentile*	50th percentile*	95th percentile*
8	1.14	1.30	1.14	1.35
9	1.22	1.42	1.22	1.46
10	1.30	1.54	1.30	1.61
11	1.40	1.68	1.44	1.75
12	1.47	1.78	1.59	1.92
13	1.61	1.96	1.70	2.07
14	1.77	2.09	1.79	2.13
15	1.86	2.21	1.88	2.21
16	1.94	2.29	1.92	2.19
17	2.00	2.34	1.96	2.25
18	2.06	2.41	1.96	2.28

* Indicates that the average boy or girl is at about this ratio; 95th% means that only 5% of boys or girls of this age have ratios this high or higher.

Most experts would suggest that people who weigh 10% above their ideal weight are overweight and people who weigh 20% to 30% over their ideal are mildly obese. Weighing 30% or more over the ideal defines obesity. Weighing 100% or more over an ideal weight is sometimes referred to as *morbid obesity*. For young people, having a very high weight–height ratio, with obviously more fat than is desired, is a problem. Calling it overweight or obesity doesn't matter. What does matter is that the odds against becoming a lean adult if you do *not* lose the weight before you reach adulthood are 28 to 1. Most overweight youngsters become overweight adults. The time to lose weight is *now*, especially if you are an overweight youngster.

Why Are You Overweight?

Why do you have a weight problem? The following four factors all play a role in this problem:

1. *Food and exercise*—the kind of food I eat, how much I exercise.
2. *Family and friends*—how my family and friends eat and exercise, their style of eating, and how important they consider eating and exercising.
3. *Emotions*—eating because I feel upset.
4. *Biology*—something being wrong with my body. I seem to gain weight faster and easier than others who seem to eat and exercise just like me.

Research has shown that being overweight is not a sign of personal weakness or neurosis. Excess weight is mainly a *biological problem* or challenge. Overcoming it requires the kind of behavioral skills needed to change one's biology — one's body. Losing weight is not the same, for most people, as trying to change the way they talk to others or the way they think about themselves. It requires changing the body in a manner very similar to the changes worked on by *highly dedicated athletes.* You need to train yourself and your body to overcome its natural tendencies. All good athletes do exactly the same thing. For example, the great football player, Walter Payton, did not have legs that "wanted" to grow to look like tree trunks; he had to *make* those changes occur through a long-term commitment and hard work.

A difficult physiology, certain family/cultural factors, and other things do *not* usually produce eating and exercising patterns that are abnormal. For examples, overweight adults usually do not eat much, if any, more than people of normal weight. The biology of obesity makes it much harder for overweight people to lose excess weight, compared with people who have never had a weight problem. So, in order to lose weight, overweight people must develop eating and exercising patterns that are abnormally difficult. These changes can be achieved, but they are supernormal. Again, remember that *losing weight is like training for athletic competition.*

How Can You Lose Weight
Safely and Permanently?

First, remember the "blame" for weight problems goes largely to your biology, not to yourself. You are *ok* (at least!); your body "simply" needs to be trained, just like an athlete's body needs to be trained. In this program, we focus on difficult and permanent changes in life-style (eating and exercising). The "training" in this program involves:

1. Learning certain self-management skills to improve your effectiveness as a "body trainer."
2. Learning to solve problems effectively.
3. Giving and receiving support, encouragement, and useful ideas with others.
4. Using the group to provide a little external pressure.

You will learn how to do all of these things step-by-step, week-by-week. Each week your group leader will introduce new ideas, help you solve problems, and ask you to write out specific goals by making a *behavioral contract*. The contract will provide you with a homework assignment for each week. The homework assignment for this week will be explained in your first meeting.

Homework

1. Both parents and children should review *and* discuss together Handout 1. Try to set aside an hour each week to do this.
2. Cut out 1 to 3 weight loss ads from newspapers or magazines and bring them in.
3. Finish the Decision Balance Sheet (Figure 2.1), following the directions provided by your group leader during the first session. Also, hang it up in a closet or on a wall and review it several times this week. Bring it back to the group for next week.
4. Start a weight graph. Be sure to include only 10 to 15 pounds on the y-axis, so you will be able to see your progress clearly. Post this graph in a place where you will see it every day (in a closet, on the inside of a door, or on a bulletin board). But weigh yourself only 1 or 2 times a week.

Chapter 3
Session 2.
Measuring Current Eating and Exercise Habits

REVIEW OF LAST WEEK'S WORK

Leader's Goal: To give clients support for progress and individual attention and help them develop an active problem-solving style.

Activities: Dyadic discussions, followed by large-group review.

Have clients talk in dyads for 10 to 20 minutes about what they did last week. Model this for them. The talks should focus on their written materials, and each client in the dyad should have 50% of the "air time." This can be done by having two children talk with each other and two parents. Group leaders should float among dyads, spending a couple of minutes with each. The dyads should review last week's work, provide support, and identify ideas and problems to be shared in the larger group. For this week, the clients should discuss their successes in achieving goals stated in contract 1, the ads they found in newspapers, their decision balance sheets, and their weight graphs. When the 10 to 20 minute dyad review is finished, bring the larger group together and discuss what each dyad learned.

COMMITMENT:
SELF-MONITORING EATING
(FROM HANDOUT 2, STEP 1)

Leader's Goal: To begin gathering data about each client's eating habits.

Activities: Review of forms, discussion.

1. Describe self-monitoring simply as accurate recording of what and where you eat, in order to discover problem areas where changes need to be made.

2. The goal for this first week of self-monitoring is just to record current eating patterns and not to change them. Emphasize to clients that they should try to eat in their usual way as much as possible this first week.
3. Review the sample parent and child Eating Diary layouts in Handout 2. Emphasize that it is very important to record *all* eating and that everyone should carry a notebook and record all eating as soon as possible after it occurs.
4. Discuss how clients now perceive their eating problems. Have them write out their predictions of where they will find problems to be reviewed next week.

SELF-MONITORING EXERCISE
(FROM LESSON 2, STEP 2)

Leader's Goal: To begin gathering data about each client's exercise habits.

Activities: Review of forms, discussion.

1. Have the clients turn to the sample exercise record. Review the Exercise and Calorie Expenditure table and Daily Exercise Record forms with the clients.
2. For next week, parent and child are to each fill out a Daily Exercise Record form and bring it in to the next session.
3. It is not necessary this first week to total up calories.
4. Discuss how and when clients currently exercise.

HOMEWORK ASSIGNMENT

Leader's Goal: To get clients thinking about and working on relevant tasks during the week.

Activities: Provision of information, including a handout; discussion of the week's tasks.

1. Parents and children are to review what happened in Session 2 and read and discuss Handout 2.
2. Parents and children are to record all eating in eating diaries.
3. Participants need to record their exercise on their own Daily Exercise Record forms.
4. Each participant would benefit from developing a positive attitude about the program and her or his likelihood of success in it.

NEW CONTRACTS

Leader's Goal: To increase compliance.

Activities: Writing and discussion of each client's new contracts.
    Include self-monitoring of food and exercise, plus reading Handout 2.

HANDOUT 2:
MEASURING CURRENT EATING
AND EXERCISE HABITS

One Step at a Time

There are several important steps in this handout that form the basis of changes you will eventually make in both your eating behavior and your life-style. Your sessions are graded and arranged in an orderly fashion. Think of the program as climbing a flight of stairs. Taking one step at a time is simple and will most certainly lead you to the top. If you try jumping from the 1st to the 10th step, you can be sure of slipping or falling back to where you started. We cannot emphasize enough the importance of progressing faithfully by taking one step of this program at a time. This stepwise approach has been successful for many, many people. A major reason for the limited success of other weight-loss programs is that they often emphasize changes that are rapid and drastic rather than the *gradual* learning of new behaviors and a new life-style. So, to be successful in the long run you must take one step at a time.

How is Eating a Problem for You?

The major task for this week is for you to identify how eating is a problem for you. Most people eat because of a wide variety of factors other than being hungry. It will be important to identify your *eating patterns* and how they keep you from losing weight.

Most people are out of touch with their eating. That is, most people do not know when and where and what they eat. For example, ask yourself how often you eat, where you eat, and with whom you eat. Your answer would probably be different from the answer given by someone who observed you during a week and made a record of your pattern of eating. You might think that you eat when you are nervous, bored, or, perhaps, depressed. This first lesson helps you develop a more specific and precise understanding of your eating patterns.

Step 1. Look Objectively at Your Eating Behavior. The first step, then, is for you to take an objective look at your eating just as an outside observer might. To say that you eat too much and exercise too little is certainly not clear enough. Your eating behavior occurs in certain specific situations. Each individual has a unique living environment and a life-style involving family, work, and a circle of friends. The purpose of this phase of the program is to determine just how your behavior and these various circumstances influence your eating. It is very important for you to identify these influences on your eating behavior in order to make use of strategies aimed at changing your eating habits. For example, if you knew the exact times of day that are most troublesome for you in regard to over-eating, then you could use this information to help control your eating.

Table 3.1. Parent's Sample Eating Diary

Martha S.

Day and Date	Food Eaten		Time (Circle if part of meal)	Social State		Where Eaten	Event Occurring Before	Mood
	Quantity	Type		Alone	With Whom			
Tuesday 11/7	8 oz 3 slices	Orange Juice White Toast w/Butter & Grape Jam	(8 a.m.)			Kitchen	Woke up	Tired
	2	Jelly Donuts	9:30 a.m.		Gail	Coffee room	Gail wanted to chat	Bored
	1	Milky Way	11:15 a.m.		Gail & Marge	Hall	Left office for break—passed candy machine	Angry at Marge
	2 slices 1 slice 2 slices 2 15 12 oz	Bologna/cheese sandwich Bologna American Cheese Rye Bread w/Mustard Small Sweet pickles Potato Chips Coke	(12:30 p.m.)		Gail, Marge, & Joan	At desk	Finished letter	Happy
	1 cup	Coffee w/1 oz Milk	3 p.m.		Joanne & Sue	Coffee room	Sitting idle at desk	Bored
	1 12 oz	Cheese Danish Coke	4:30 p.m.		Marge	At desk	Marge asked if I wanted a Coke	Anxious

Table 3.1. Parent's Sample Eating Diary (continued)

Martha S.

Day and Date	Food Eaten Quantity	Type	Time (Circle if part of meal)	Social State Alone	With Whom	Where Eaten	Event Occurring Before	Mood
	1	Broiled Chicken Leg	(6 p.m.)		Husband	Kitchen & living room for dessert	Came home from work and prepared dinner	Tired
	1/2 cup	Broccoli w/Butter						
	1 med.	Baked Potato w/Sour Cream						
	1 cup	Coffee w/1 oz Milk						
	2	Donuts						
	1 cup	Vanilla Fudge Ice Cream	9:30 p.m.		Husband	Living Room w/TV	Jack got some ice cream	Tired & Bored
Wednesday	8 oz	Orange Juice	(7:45 a.m.)			Kitchen	Woke up early	Tired
	1 cup	Coffee w/1 oz Milk						
	3	Donuts						
	1	Hot Dog & Roll w/Mustard & Sauerkraut	(12:30 p.m.)		Other secretaries	Cafeteria	Finished a busy morning's work	Busy
	12 oz	Coke						
	1 med.	Apple						
	2 cup	Spag. w/Meat Sauce	(6:30 p.m.)		Husband	Kitchen	Came home from work	Relaxed
	2 med.	Meatballs						
	2 in.	Ital. Bread w/Butter						
	4 oz	Red Wine						
	1 cup.	Salad w/Oil & Vinegar						
	2 in. wedge	Banana Cake w/Icing	11 p.m.		Husband	In Bed	Passed refrig. on way to bed	Tired

Table 3.2. Sample Child's Eating Diary

Peggy M.

Day of Week and Date	Food Eaten		Time (Circle if part of meal)	Where Eaten
	Amount	Type of Food		
Wednesday 3/11	5 oz	Orange Juice	(7:30 a.m.)	Kitchen
	2 oz	Cheerios w/Milk & Sugar		
	8 oz	Milk		
		Hamburger:	(12:30 p.m.)	School Cafeteria
	1 small	HB Meat		
	1	Bun		
	2	Pickles		
		Ketchup		
	1/2 cup	Jello		
	8 oz	Chocolate Milk		
	1	Milky Way Candy Bar	12:45 p.m.	Candy Machine
	8	Chocolate Chip Cookies	3:30 p.m.	Living Room w/TV
	2 pieces	Fried Chicken	(6 p.m.)	Dining Room
	1 med	Baked Potato w/ Butter		
	1/2 cup	Peas w/Butter		
	8 oz	Milk		
	1 cup	Chocolate Ice Cream		
	4	Chocolate Chip Cookies	8:30 p.m.	Living Room w/TV

For this first step, then, you need to observe your eating. Use an Eating Diary similar to the ones in Tables 3.1 and 3.2 and carry your diary with you at all times. Each time food is eaten, you are to list in your Eating Diary all of the following details:

Parent
1. Date and day
2. Food eaten — quantity and type
3. Time (circle if part of a meal)
4. Social state — alone or with others
5. Where the food was eaten
6. The event occurring immediately prior to eating
7. Your mood at the time of eating

Child
1. Date and day
2. Food eaten — quantity and type
3. Time (circle if part of a meal)
4. Where the food was eaten

Tables 3.1 and 3.2 are sample layouts for both parent's and child's eating diaries. The parent sample information was collected by Martha S., a 32-year-old secretary. Included in Martha's record of Tuesday and Wednesday is all the food she ate at meals and snacks. Notice that Martha's records were very specific. She had a bologna and cheese sandwich on Tuesday for lunch that was made of two slices of bologna, one slice of cheese, two slices of rye bread and mustard. With it she had two small sweet pickles, 15 potato chips, and a 12 oz can of Coke. The specifics of eating are very important. Recording just a bologna sandwich would not have provide Martha S. the details she needed to analyze her eating habits carefully.

The child sample information was collected by Peggy M., a 10-year-old girl. Again, note how carefully Peggy kept her records. (For some items, it might be necessary for the parent to help the child estimate the size of food portions.)

You should carry your Eating Diary with you at all times. Have it nearby, so you can write down the food you ate as soon as possible after eating it. Women might want to keep their diaries in their purses, and men should be able to fit their diaries into their back pockets. Ideally, you should record your eating immediately after each meal or snack. If it is inconvenient to record soon after eating, you should arrange to record it as soon as circumstances permit. The longer you postpone recording, the greater the chance of not doing an accurate job or of forgetting altogether. Remember, *if you have the time to eat something, make the time to record it!*

During this second week of the program, you should eat as you have in the past. Make no attempt at this point to change your eating in the slightest manner. You might notice a tendency to eat less as a result of keeping the record. Although this is okay, you should try, as much as possible, to eat the foods you usually eat in amounts and times that are typical for you.

Step 2. Keep Track of Your Exercise Level. The second step in this lesson is for you both to keep track of your exercise and activity level over the next week. Review the Exercise and Calorie Expenditure form (Figure 3.1). It classifies common exercises and activities into light, moderate, or heavy exercise. Also, for the next week, both parents and children should record any exercise or physical activity done for *at least 5 minutes* on the Daily Exercise Record form (Figure 3.2). You should each use a separate Daily Exercise Record form. Remember, this exercise or activity does not need to be an organized exercise to be included. Walking to school or to a store are excellent exercises and should be included on the forms. Use the Exercise and Calorie Expenditure Handout to classify the

FIGURE 3.1. Exercise and Calorie Expenditure Handout

Light Exercise (4 calories per minute)
Dancing (slow)
Gardening (light)
Golf
Table tennis
Volleyball
Walking (3 miles per hour)
Bowling
Downhill Skiing
Canoeing
Throwing horseshoes
Lawn mowing (power)
Horseback riding
Bicycling (5 miles per hour)

Moderate Exercise (7 calories per minute)
Badminton
Bicycling (9.5 miles per hour)
Dancing (fast)
Gardening (heavy)
Stationary cycling (moderate)
Swimming (30 yds per minute)
Tennis
Walking (4.5 miles per hour)
Ice skating, Roller skating
Cross-country skiing
Calisthenics (moderate)

Heavy Exercise (10 Calories per minute)
Calisthenics (fast)
Climbing stairs (up and down)
Bicycling (12 miles per hour)
Handball, paddleball, squash
Jogging
Skipping rope
Stationary cycling (fast)
Stationary jogging
Swimming (40 yds per minute)
Basketball

exercise or activity as light, moderate, or heavy, and check the appropriate box. Be sure to include the number of minutes of exercise. For this week, adding up the number of calories used is optional. A sample Daily Exercise Record form for Barbara T., a 12-year-old girl, is included (Figure 3.3).

FIGURE 3.2. Daily Exercise Record

Day	Exercise	L (4)	M (7)	H (10)	No. of Min.	Calories Used Up
1						
2						
3						
4						
5						
6						
7						

Week of _____ through _____ Name _____

Total calories used up this week: _____

Step 3. Develop a Positive Attitude. The last and perhaps most important step in this handout is to develop a positive attitude toward yourself and your progress. Developing a positive attitude early in the program is necessary, because it is well known that how you think about yourself can have a very powerful influence on your behavior. Thus, if you start the program believing that you will fail, you will reduce your chances for success. So, where does this lead you? First, it will be important for you to change the way you think about yourself. It

FIGURE 3.3. Daily Exercise Record

Week of __3/10__ through __3/16__					Name __Barbara T.__	
Day	Exercise	L (4)	M (7)	H (10)	No. of Min.	Calories Used Up
1 Wed.	Walked to and from school	X			20	80
2 Thurs.	Walked to school	X			10	40
	Gymnastics		X		30	210
3 Fri.						
4 Sat.	Rode bicycle	X			20	80
5 Sun.						
6 Mon.	Walked to and from school	X			20	80
7 Tues.	Walked to and from school	X			20	80
				Total calories used up this week:		570

is helpful *not* to think of yourself as a person who is permanently stuck in a fat body. You can begin to relate your overweight condition to your behavior and the way you live. In fact, current research indicates that when people make big changes in how they eat and exercise, they can lose weight. When you think of your overweight condition in this manner, it is clear what changes need to be made. That is, you can focus on changing your eating behavior and activity patterns. This is exactly what you will be doing throughout this program.

As you progress through the program, you will probably experience something that many who have gone before you have noticed. That is, there will be a tendency to think in statements such as "I'm basically a fat person." This negative attitude, or thought, will arise particularly during difficult times. If you accept that you are basically a fat person, you are accepting a false idea. This amounts to admitting defeat, giving yourself an easy cop-out. To overcome this negative tendency, it helps to recognize these negative thoughts, label them as false, and prevent yourself from falling into the trap of saying again that you are basically a fat person.

You might feel that the tasks set forward in this handout are very simple and easy to do. The program is planned that way, and the steps to follow are equally easy to carry out. The difficulty involved in progressing through this program is one of making the initial decision to start it and to take control of the circumstances that affect your eating and exercising. Once you have decided to follow this program, it can be your companion and provide helpful assistance for years.

This handout does not require you to change your eating behavior or to increase your exercise. It merely asks you to observe as closely as possible your eating behavior, the situations in which it occurs, and what precedes the act of eating. In other words, this session asks you to define as closely as possible the problem that eating represents for you. The steps are relatively easy, although they require commitment on your part. Remember: The information you gather this week will be crucial to your future success.

Homework

1. Review with your child what happened at Session 2 as soon as possible after the session is over.
2. Read Handout 2 carefully. Encourage your child to read it too, discussing any parts that are difficult for him or her to understand.
3. Record *all* eating in your eating diaries.
4. Record all exercise on a Daily Exercise Record form (parent and child are to use separate forms).
5. Develop a positive attitude toward yourself and your progress.

Remember to bring all materials to the next session!

Chapter 4
Session 3.
Beginning to Change

REVIEW OF LAST WEEK'S WORK

Leader's Goal: To help reinforce progress, provide attention, and identify problems.

Activities: Dyadic discussions, followed by large-group discussion.

See if any problems arose last week in self-monitoring of eating or exercise. If anyone brings up problems, try to see if the group can come up with ideas first before answering the questions yourself.

STIMULUS CONTROL

Leader's Goal: To reduce the number of stimuli that clients associate with eating.

Activities: Dyadic discussion and completion of Meal Schedule sheets.

Discussion

"What we are going to do is to start to break the connection between things around you and your eating. Three techniques can help you do this."

1. *Limit Eating*

   The first step is to try to begin eating *three, and only three, meals a day*, plus an afternoon snack for a child. Clients are allowed to eat as much as they need at each meal, in order to make this step as easy as possible.

   Between meals, they can have as many "free" foods as desired. These include (a) black coffee (parents only), (b) plain or herb tea, (c) diet soda, (d) sugarless gum, (e) bouillon (*Caution:* Too much bouillon can cause temporary water retention because of its high salt content).

2. *Schedule Meals in Advance*

    Clients are to use their Meal Schedules (see Figures 4.1 and 4.2) to plan *when* and *where* their meals are to be eaten next week. If possible, clients should try to schedule meals at the same time and place each day. Have parents and children work together for a few minutes planning their meals for next week and filling out their Meal Schedule sheets.

3. *Monitor Extra Snacks*

    (a) Any eating other than planned meals is to be recorded in the clients' eating diaries as usual. In addition, they are to mark a big XS next to it, designating as an *Extra Snack*.

    (b) For the next week, although clients should try to limit extra snacking as much as they can, the important thing is to *record all* extra snacks in their diaries.

    (c) It is *important* to emphasize to the clients that extra snacking is *not* an indication of failure and instead only points out an area that needs more work in the future.

Summary of Stimulus Control

Emphasize to the clients that:

1. They are not giving up any food they like.
2. They can eat as much as they want.
3. They are learning *skills* that allow them to establish self-control over their eating habits.

STOPPERS

Leader's Goal: To help clients cope with urges to eat by engaging in incompatible behaviors.

Activities: Review of forms, discussion.

Discussion

A *stopper* is something you can do when you are feeling bored or hungry that will reduce your desire to eat or make it difficult for you to eat. Some examples might be chewing gum, playing outside, riding your bicycle, working on a project, and doing household chores.

Group Activity

Have clients pair up (pair parent with his or her own child for this exercise) and talk to each other about possible ideas for stoppers. After a few minutes, have people share some of their ideas and write them on a blackboard.

Homework

Refer clients to their Stoppers Worksheets (Handout 3). For the next week, they are each to make up a list of from 10 to 15 stoppers and write them down on their worksheets.

EXERCISE

Leader's Goal: To encourage clients to exercise.

Activity: Completion of exercise-planning sheets.

Discussion

Give a *short* talk on exercise, how important it is in a weight-control program and so on, from Handout 3. Talk about desirable kinds of exercise such as walking, swimming, jogging, and tennis versus less useful kinds of exercise such as sit-ups and jumping jacks.

For next week, parent and child are to *increase* their exercise and activity levels by a total of 750 calories burned up over the week. We recommend that parent and child try to do at least some exercise together. *They must exercise at least once every other day.*

Group Activity

Have the parent and her or his child pair up and plan their exercise for next week, recording their plans on their Weekly Exercise Planning Worksheets (See Figure 4.4 in Handout 3).

Homework

1. Complete the Weekly Exercise Planning Worksheets for next week, if not done during the session. These worksheets are to be posted in a prominent place at home, for example on bedroom walls.
2. Record daily exercise on the Daily Exercise Record sheets, including the number of calories burned up. Beginning this week, clients should only record new exercise toward their weekly exercise goal. The Daily Exercise Record sheets should be posted on the wall next to their Planning Worksheets, as reminders of their exercise plans for the week.
3. Mark the total calories burned up each day on the Daily Exercise Graphs.
4. At the end of the week, mark the total calories burned up for the week on a combined Weekly Exercise Graph.

HOMEWORK ASSIGNMENT

Leader's Goal: To get clients thinking about and working on relevant tasks during the week.

Activities: Provision of information and a handout, discussion of the week's tasks.

1. Parents and children are to review and discuss Session 3.
2. Participants are to complete and post Weekly Exercise Planning worksheets.
3. Clients are to complete Meal Schedules.
4. Parents should aim for three meals per day, whereas children aim for three meals per day and one afternoon snack.
5. Clients should mark extra snacks XS in eating diaries.
6. Participants are to complete stoppers worksheets.
7. Parents and children are to begin an exercise program with a 750-calorie expenditure as a goal.
8. Clients are to complete weekly Exercise Graphs.
9. Parents and children are to continue self-monitoring food and working on positive attitudes.

NEW CONTRACT

Leader's Goal: To increase compliance.

Activity: Completion of new contracts.

Include stimulus control suggestions, development of lists of stoppers, self-monitoring of food and exercise, and exercise goal.

HANDOUT 3:
BEGINNING TO CHANGE

This week we will begin the process of making gradual changes in your eating habits and activity patterns. But, before we begin these new topics, let's review the steps presented in Handout 2.

Look at your eating diaries. Were there *any* meals or snacks not recorded? If so, remember that it is crucial to record *all* of your eating in the future. Completely recording all of your eating is the only way you can be sure of what you have eaten and what you need to change.

Did you record all of your exercise or other physical activity? Does your Daily Exercise Record show a log of physical activity or just a little? For most overweight people, their Daily Exercise Records for the first week do not show a lot of physical activity. We will be focusing on the importance of exercise in your weight-control program later in this lesson.

The last major topic from last week was to work on developing a positive attitude toward yourself. Did you catch yourself thinking any negative thoughts such as "I'm basically a fat person and just won't ever be able to change?" As you progress through this program, it should become much easier for you to combat these negative thoughts, because you will be able to see clearly that you *can* change because you *will be* changing your eating and exercising patterns!

Now let's go on to the new topics for this week. These include *shaping, deprivation*, and *stimulus control*. These terms might be new to you. The words are simply labels used to describe principles of behavior that you will use in this program. Each term will be fully explained to you in this session by reference to common examples.

Shaping

Shaping is a process of inching toward permanent changes in behavior. Remember that each step in the program is designed to approximate one step on a flight of stairs. Making such gradual changes can help you maintain change over a long period of time. Thus, permanent changes in eating are accomplished best in a very gradual manner. Small changes, when they accumulate, lead to more appropriate behavior and weight loss.

There are many examples of shaping in our daily lives. Children, for instance, must be taught to add and subtract before they can go on to more difficult arithmetic problems such as multiplication and division. In the same way, teaching a child to talk or to say a simple word such as *daddy* involves a shaping process. Initially, the child will say *da-da* and then gradually *d-d*. Eventually, with the parents as shapers, the child will be able to combine the *da* and *d* into "Daddy." Likewise, a beginning musician learns to play the piano by striking one key at a time. Chords are then mastered, and eventually the building up of these basic skills bit by bit enables the pianist to play more complex music.

In this program, the desired goals and behaviors are eating and activity patterns that will maintain an ideal weight. It takes time. Advancing in small steps will assure that you gradually learn more appropriate patterns. The chances of acquiring and maintaining desired goal behaviors over a long period of time would be small if you attempted to adopt them too quickly. Therefore, the principle of shaping used in this program is a means by which the final eating behaviors can be acquired gradually and permanently.

Deprivation

Deprivation refers to the tendency to be hungry as the time lengthens since your last meal. Generally, as the time without food increases, there is a greater tendency to eat. You have probably tried one or more of the popular diets that restrict either calorie intake or the type of food you can eat. Many of these diets are very difficult to maintain over a long period of time. That is because as you deprive yourself of either calories or foods that you like, the tendency to break your diet increases. This is one reason why these diets are failures. A good dieter will stick to the crash program for several days. Perhaps a more determined individual is even able to maintain the discipline for up to 1 or 2 weeks. However, individuals rarely remain on these diets for 3 or more weeks. In this program, we expect that you will make relatively few dramatic shifts in the kinds of food you eat. If you like pizza or potatoes, we expect that you will be able to eat these and still lose weight. What you will learn, however, is where, when, how, and in what amounts to eat these items. This program does not advise, at least at this stage, specific calorie reductions or deviations from your preferred foods. You are to minimize food deprivation and thereby decrease the tendency to overeat.

Stimulus Control

Stimulus control is a term that refers to the relationship between eating and the situations in which eating occurs. For example, the TV commercials for hamburgers might send you to the refrigerator. Preparing a meal in the kitchen might get you to nibble on the food you are preparing. The smell from a bakery shop might make you want to stop and buy some cookies. Even the clock striking noon could be associated with lunchtime and influence you to eat. Generally, research indicates that the eating behavior of overweight individuals, more so than normally weighted individuals, is influenced by external stimuli such as these. That is, the features of the environment such as the time of day, other individuals' eating, food ads, and even the mere sight of food initiate eating in overweight individuals. Normal-sized persons, however, do not respond as much to these external food cues.

Look at your Eating Diary. You might notice that there are certain situations that seem for you to be very closely associated with eating. Many of these situations are inappropriate for eating. It is necessary to break the association between these inappropriate situations and your eating behavior. You will use the idea of stimulus control to decrease the number of inappropriate situations in which you eat.

Step 1. Decreasing Eating Situations. The first step for this week is to decrease the number of situations in which eating occurs. Review your diary. Aren't there many different situations in which your eating has occurred? As a first step in limiting the way situations control your eating, you (the parent) will begin to eat three and *only three meals per day,* and your child will begin to eat *only three meals per day plus an afternoon snack.* All food intake should occur only during these three meals (plus snack for the child). The importance of this task cannot be emphasized enough. This might seem like an impossible chore, but read on. We will describe exactly how you can do it.

Step 2. Scheduling Meals. As soon as possible, both of you should fill out the Parent's and Child's Meal Schedules (Figures 4.1 and 4.2). It helps if you schedule your meals at the same time and place every day. However, try not to schedule meals too late in the evening, because this will leave little time to digest your food

FIGURE 4.1. Parent's Meal Schedule

Day	Meal	Time	Place
Week of _____ thru _____ Name _____			
	Breakfast		
	Lunch		
	Dinner		
	Breakfast		
	Lunch		
	Dinner		
	Breakfast		
	Lunch		
	Dinner		
	Breakfast		
	Lunch		
	Dinner		
	Breakfast		
	Lunch		
	Dinner		
	Breakfast		
	Lunch		
	Dinner		
	Breakfast		
	Lunch		
	Dinner		

prior to going to bed. Try to anticipate when and where you will be eating. The whole idea of stimulus control is that it helps you to plan and control when you eat rather than letting your environment and certain situations control your eating. The presence of others, access to the refrigerator, food ads, and so on, should no longer control your eating.

If you eat at times not indicated in your meal schedule or you eat more than

FIGURE 4.2. Child's Meal Schedule

Week of _____ thru _____ Name _____			
Day	Meal	Time	Place
	Breakfast		
	Lunch		
	Snack		
	Dinner		
	Breakfast		
	Lunch		
	Snack		
	Dinner		
	Breakfast		
	Lunch		
	Snack		
	Dinner		
	Breakfast		
	Lunch		
	Snack		
	Dinner		
	Breakfast		
	Lunch		
	Snack		
	Dinner		
	Breakfast		
	Lunch		
	Snack		
	Dinner		
	Breakfast		
	Lunch		
	Snack		
	Dinner		

three meals (plus snack for the child) a day, this should be labeled and recorded in your diary as an "extra snack" and marked *XS*. In your diary put *XS* next to any eating that does not occur during your planned meals. Most important is that episodes of extra snacking are *not* an indication of failure. In other *diet* programs, once you break the diet, you go off it entirely. Not so with our program; you merely record the extra snacking and learn to control it.

Step 3. Limiting Extra Snacking. For this next week, we want you to make an effort to limit extra snacking, but we will not give you a specified goal. What is important for now is to carefully keep track of your extra snacking in your Eating Diary. Be sure to circle the times that indicate a planned meal or snack so that *XSs* will be very apparent to you as you continue to analyze your eating behaviors.

There are certain "free" foods you may have any time without recording them as extra snacks. For parents, they include black coffee, plain tea, herbal tea, and bouillon. For children, they include diet soda, sugarless gum, and bouillon. They also include most raw vegetables such as celery, carrots, and sour pickles. Thus, if you need something in addition to the planned meals, use a free food to tide you over until the next meal. Also, to decrease the effect of deprivation, you should eat as much as you like during the planned meals. You will be decreasing the amount you eat later, but, for now, this step emphasizes your ability to regulate and plan meals. Try to limit the occasions for eating to just the planned times each day. No other food should be eaten between meals other than the few free foods listed. It is not the calories you are worried about now but achieving stimulus control.

Let's review some of the ideas we have talked about under the topics of stimulus control and deprivation. Try to remember that (a) you are not giving up eating, (b) you are to eat the foods that you like, and (c) you can eat as much as you want to. The changes you will be making in this third period are limited to the planning and programming of your eating. By doing this, you are changing the conditions under which you are eating and beginning to establish control over your food intake, rather than letting it occur on the basis of uncontrolled influences.

Step 4. Focusing on Feelings of Hunger. Feelings of hunger and deprivation will probably occur occasionally during this program. If you feel hungry, that is great! Focus on that feeling. Notice the hunger pangs. Try to make this a very, very positive experience. As we mentioned earlier, the eating behavior of overweight people is often under the control of external features such as the time of day or the sight of food. Feelings of hunger are internal stimuli, which are most helpful in telling you when you are hungry. Think of them as fantastic! You should feel good about being hungry. There is nothing wrong with feeling hungry. You know from your meal schedule when and where you will eat your next meal.

Hunger, then, is a very positive experience in two ways. *First*, you are becoming sensitive to feelings in your body and thus becoming less of a slave to your environment. *Second,* you can recognize that if you do experience hunger pangs, this means that there is nothing available in your stomach. Your body must then go to the available fat stores to provide its energy requirements. The discomfort associated with hunger pangs is temporary. Notice the hunger pangs, feel good about them, and don't worry—they won't kill you. Feel sure that your body is using up excess fatty tissue.

Feelings of hunger should be closely linked with food deprivation. After several days on three planned meals, your body will begin to conform to the new schedule. Feelings of hunger, stomach growls, and such will be more evident just before mealtime. This is true hunger and different from the vague desires to eat to which you are probably used to responding.

Step 5. Identifying Stoppers. The next step in this week's work is to make up a list of special activities that we call *stoppers.* A stopper is simply an activity that will interfere with your desire to eat or will interrupt ongoing eating. Activities that are incompatible with eating, such as chewing gum, playing outside, running, building models, and doing house cleaning are classified as stoppers. Notice that it is either difficult or almost impossible to eat while engaging in an activity labeled a stopper. To qualify as a stopper , again, the activity should be incompatible with eating, but it should also be something you can readily begin. Once you have begun a stopper, it should be difficult to stop. If you enjoy the activity, so much the better, although chores often meet the requirements for a stopper.

For next week, both parents and children are to make a list of 10 to 15 stoppers and write them down on their Stoppers Worksheet (Figure 4.3). In our next handout, we will discuss how to use stoppers to help reduce extra snacking. For this week, however, we are only asking you to prepare your list of stoppers.

FIGURE 4.3. Stoppers Worksheet

Name _____

In the space below, write down 10 to 15 things you could do instead of snacking when you are feeling bored or hungry. These activities should be things that make it hard for you to eat while you are doing them.

Exercise

Work and activity require energy, which is supplied by the food we eat. So, food is the fuel for our bodies. When your output of energy does not utilize all the fuel you consume, the extra fuel is stored as fat. This serves several positive functions. The stored fat supplies a source of energy for later use, keeps you warm, provides padding, and is the basis of a desirable body shape. However, as you know, when this process is carried to an extreme, it can result in an overweight condition.

Today our life is full of conveniences that require us to do less and less physical work. You can go just about anywhere with little or no walking. Household chores such as cleaning and food preparation demand little physical work. Most occupations have also profited from technical advances, and now there is little in the way of physical labor. The typical worker just sits behind a desk or operates machinery. It is an established fact that overweight is more common in those whose work requires little activity. This association of overweight and inactivity is true for all ages. Heavier infants are less active. The same is true for adolescents and adults. It is precisely this association of inactivity and overweight that makes exercise such an important component of our program.

Many studies have shown that lack of activity, in addition to overeating, is a likely cause of overweight. The action of obese laboratory animals, which consists mainly of eating, supports this. They eat, then immediately sleep. Upon their awakening, the cycle of sleeping and eating continues. In fact, it is very difficult to breed these animals successfully because they will not expend the necessary energy to reproduce. Let's take an example from animal husbandry. Most livestock are "fattened up" prior to sale on the market. The animals are placed in very small pens to restrict their movement. In addition to having free access to food, these animals expend little energy. Their eating actually increases as the area in which they live becomes confined and restricted.

Therefore, the last step in this lesson involves increasing your physical activity. You and your child are to begin a regular exercise program, planning some activity to do at home but also utilizing programs available in the community such as your public school system or YMCA.

Step 6. Surveying Exercise Resources. The first step in regard to your exercise program will be for you to survey the resources in your community. Look in the newspaper, contact friends, and call the YMCA or the YWCA. Find out what types of exercise programs are available in your area.

There are so many positive things to say about exercise that it is hard to begin. *First*, you will find that it goes hand in hand with controlling your eating behavior. One seems to encourage the other. As you start to gain effective control over your eating behavior, it will be easier to manage your exercise. *Second*, the energy expended through exercise is a valuable adjunct to weight reduction through your changes in eating. Our research shows that those who exercise regularly, besides becoming physically fit, have the greatest weight loss over a one-year period. Your body size and your passive life-style might make you feel reluctant to undertake an exercise program. Be assured that as you increase your exercise and energy expenditure, you will begin to feel very good, even great! Just as you will begin to notice hunger feelings in your stomach, a regular exercise program will also make you aware of other feelings in your body.

As with food, we recommend no specific exercise, and you should do things that you were accustomed to and enjoyed in the past. If, for example, you used to bowl, ice skate, or play tennis, take it up again. Generally, the best forms of exercise are those that involve regular movement over a period of time and that use many muscle groups in a coordinated fashion. The two best examples of these exercises, which we call *rhythmic exercise*, are swimming and jogging. Walking is also an excellent exercise. Calisthenics such as jumping jacks, push-ups, toe touches, and sit-ups, although not rhythmic in nature, increase muscle tone and are recommended as warm-ups prior to rhythmic activity.

Remember, however, it is the rhythmic exercise that best increases muscle tone, improves the heart and lung functions, and expends energy. You might want to look at Dr. Cooper's *The New Aerobics*, Jim Fixx's *The Complete Book of Running*, or Dr. Shehan's *On Running* for examples of good exercise programs. Regardless of what you do, try to make it as much fun as possible. Exercising with others is great fun! It is our experience that exercise can be not only fun, but the most rewarding part of this program. If exercise is new to you, begin with a nonstrenuous program, such as walking, and gradually increase it to include more strenuous activity.

Step 7. Increasing Fitness and Burning up Calories. Beginning this week, you and your child are each to expend a *total of 750 calories* through increased exercise. This energy expenditure should be *in addition* to any exercise or activity you normally engage in. If you now walk to work or school, for example, all well and good, but you can't count it as additional energy expenditure.

It is important that you do some exercise *at least every other day*, rather than try to expend the entire 750 calories in 1 or 2 days. Plan your exercise so it fits into your general routine. Make it part of your life. Establishment of an active life-style is one of the most important components of this program.

Because a major emphasis of this program is on you and your child's working together, try to make at least part of your exercise plans something you and your child can do *together*. Some possibilities might include walking, jogging, bicycling, playing tennis, and swimming.

Each week you and your child should work together planning your exercise for the next week. Use the Weekly Exercise Planning Worksheet (Figure 4.4) to record these plans. Because this exercise is to be *in addition* to your normal activity level, it is usually easier to just include your new activities on the worksheet. That is, if you walk to work each day, it is not necessary to include it in your plans for next week, because it will not count toward your weekly increased energy expenditure goal.

FIGURE 4.4. Weekly Exercise Planning Worksheet

Week of _____ thru _____　　　　　Name _____

Day	Exercise	Where	When	L (4)	M (7)	H (10)	# of Min.	Calories Used Up

Total Calories Planned This Week: _____

Goal For This Week: _____

When filling out your Weekly Exercise Planning Worksheets, it is very important to fill in the columns labeled "Where" and "When." The more detailed your plans, the easier they are to follow. In addition, it is very desirable to try to plan your activities at the same time each day whenever possible. For example, if you plan to jog on Monday, Wednesday, and Friday next week, it is better to plan to jog at the *same time* on each of these days. After you have completed your Planning Worksheets for next week, post them in a prominent place such as on the walls in your bedrooms or in the bathroom.

Step 8. Monitoring your Exercise Each Day. At the end of each day, you and your child should record your exercise for the day on your Daily Exercise Record forms (included in Handout 2). It is only necessary to keep track of your increased exercise, which counts toward your goal this week of 750 calories. Be sure to record the number of minutes of exercise; classify it as Light, Moderate, or Heavy exercise; and record the number of calories burned up.

Once you have completed recording your exercise for the day, total up the calories burned up and mark this figure on your Daily Exercise Graph. (If your child has trouble understanding this, you will have to help him or her fill out the Daily and Weekly Exercise Graphs.) You and your child should post your Daily Exercise Graphs in prominent places to help you remember to do your exercise and record it daily. A good place to put it is right next to your Weekly Exercise Planning Worksheet so you can see how well you are following your plan for the week.

Step 9. Monitoring your Exercise at the End of the Week. At the end of the week, you and your child are to add up the total number of calories burned up through exercise and record these totals on your combined Weekly Exercise Graph. The goals for each week of the program are marked on this graph, so you can easily check your progress over the entire course of this program.

As was mentioned earlier, exercise can be an effective inhibitor of eating. There is a myth, however, that exercise increases appetite. On the contrary, exercise often *decreases* appetite; so rather than increasing your feelings of hunger, exercising will decrease them.

There are two important features of the exercise program that we must emphasize, one being psychological, the other being medical. A regular exercise program will decrease feelings of tension and help you function more efficiently in a wide variety of activities. Right after you exercise, take 5 or 10 minutes to sit and relax. You will find that this cooling down period is very refreshing and enjoyable. The other set of benefits, medical, is also very important. A regular exercise program will increase your circulation and improve a variety of functions, including those of your heart, kidneys, and lungs. It will tone up your body muscles and make you more aware of and in touch with your body.

Step 10. Thinking Positively. At the start of each day, you should look over your meal schedules. Remember to anticipate when and where you will be eating. Also, recall the changes you have made in your eating and exercise to this point and feel good about these gains. You should feel yourself engaging in a continuous pattern of change and concentrate on the positive future ahead.

Homework

New Tasks This Week

1. Review together what happened at Session 3 as soon as possible after the session is over.
2. Plan together your exercise for next week and record your plans on your Weekly Exercise Planning Worksheets. Post these worksheets on your bedroom wall or some other easy-to-see place.
3. Fill out your Meal Schedules for next week. Try to eat at the same time each day.
4. (Parent) Restrict your eating to three meals a day.
   (Child) Restrict your eating to three meals a day plus an afternoon snack.
5. Mark any extra snacks (excluding free foods) *XS* in your Eating Diaries.
6. Make up a list of 10 to 15 stoppers and record them on your Stoppers Worksheets.
7. Begin your exercise program. The goal for next week is an increase of 750 calories burned up. Each day record your exercise on your Daily Exercise Records and your Daily Exercise Graphs.
8. At the end of the week, record the total calories burned up on your combined Weekly Exercise Graph.

Continued Tasks

1. Record *all* eating (except free foods) in your Eating Diaries.
2. Develop a positive attitude toward yourself and your progress.

Remember to bring in all materials to the next session!

Chapter 5
Session 4.
Food, Nutrition, and Weight

REVIEW OF LAST WEEK'S WORK

Leader's Goal: To help reinforce progress, provide attention, and identify problems.

Activities: Dyadic discussions, followed by large-group discussion.

When large group reconvenes, briefly discuss problems with last week's work. Some issues that come up could be discussed when the relevant topic arises this week (e.g., stoppers, stimulus control, exercise).

NUTRITION

Leader's Goal: To help client's improve the nutritional quality of their diets.

Activities: Completion of a checklist measuring the nutritional adequacy of one day's eating, discussion.

Discussion

Briefly review the nutritional information in the handouts (e.g., the 4 food groups from Table 5.1). Answer any questions that arise. If you don't know an answer, check a sourcebook like Brody (1981).

Group Activity

Ask participants to turn to Table 5.1. Hand out copies of Figures 5.1 and 5.2. Review Figure 5.1 and discuss how it was completed. Then have each pair of participants (e.g., each parent–child dyad) complete one Figure 5.2 based on a review of one of their recent day's self-monitoring records. Help the dyads do this by going from dyad to dyad and discussing their work as they try to complete it.

Table 5.1. Servings in the Basic Four Food Groups

Food	Amount per serving*	Servings per day
	Milk Group	
Milk	8 oz (1 cup)	Children 0–9 years: 2 to 3
Yogurt, plain	1 cup	Children 9–12 years: 3
Hard cheese	1¼ oz	Teens: 4
Cheese spread	2 oz	Adults: 2
Ice cream	1½ cups	Pregnant women: 3
Cottage cheese	2 cups	Nursing mothers: 4
	Meat Group	
Meat, lean	2 to 3 oz, cooked	2 (can be eaten as mixtures of
Poultry	2 to 3 oz	animal and vegetable foods; if
Fish	2 to 3 oz	only vegetable protein is
Hard cheese	2 to 3 oz	consumed, it must be
Eggs	2 to 3	balanced)
Cottage cheese	½ cup	
Dry beans and peas	1 to 1½ cups cooked	
Nuts and seeds	½ to ¾ cup	
Peanut butter	4 tablespoons	
	Vegetable and Fruit Group	
Vegetables, cut up	½ cup	4, including one good vitamin
Fruits, cut up	½ cup	C source such as oranges or
Grapefruit	½ medium	orange juice and one
Melon	½ medium	deep-yellow or dark-green
Orange	1	vegetable
Potato	1 medium	
Salad	1 bowl	
Lettuce	1 wedge	
	Bread and Cereal Group	
Bread	1 slice	4, whole grain or enriched
Cooked cereal	½ to ¾ cup	only, including at least one
Pasta	½ to ¾ cup	serving of whole grain
Rice	½ to ¾ cup	
Dry cereal	1 oz	

* These amounts were established by the U.S. Department of Agriculture to meet specific nutritional requirements. For the milk group, serving size is based on the calcium content of 1 cup of milk. For the meat group, serving size is determined by the protein content. Thus, rather than eat 2 cups of cottage cheese (milk group) or 4 tbs of peanut butter (meat group), it would make more sense to eat half those amounts and count each as half a serving in their respective groups. If cottage cheese (½ cup) is consumed as a meat substitute, you may count it as a full meat serving and a quarter of a milk serving.

Bring the group back together and ask them to discuss any deficiencies they discovered. Many of their diets will be high on the meat group and low on the vegetable and fruit group. For those with clear deficiencies, have them set specific nutritional changes as goals for this week's contract.

FIGURE 5.1. 1-Day Sample of a Food Diary, Checked for Nutritional Quality

Time	Food (Specific Amount)	Milk Group	Meat Group	Vegetable & Fruit Group	Bread & Cereal Group
				Servings in Food Groups	
8 AM	Shredded wheat cereal 1.5 ozs				1.5
	Skim milk 1 cup	1			
12 Noon	Cheese sandwich:				
	4 ozs Cheese		2		
	.5 Lettuce wedge			.5	
	.25 cup Tomato			.5	
	2 slices Bread				2
3 PM	Snack:				
	¼ cup Peanuts		.5		
	2 Chocolate cookies	—	—	—	—
	1 glass Skim milk	1			
6 PM	Salad (1 bowl)			1	
	6 ozs Steak		2		
	2 medium Potatoes			2	
	½ cup Green beans			1	
10 PM	3 cups Popcorn			1	
Totals:		2	4.5	6	3.5
Recommended Totals (for Adults):		2	2	4	4
Adequacy (0 = at requirement; + = met or exceeded requirement; - = below requirement)		0	+ 2.5	+ 2	-.5

CALORIES AND WEIGHT

Leader's Goal: To improve understanding of energy balance and the importance of self-monitoring calories.

Activity: Use of a calorie-counting book to look up calories of fast foods and alternative meals.

FIGURE 5.2. Nutritional Checklist Form for One Day's Eating
(See Table 5.1 for definitions of serving sizes for each food group)

		Servings in Food Groups			
Time	Food (Specific Amount)	Milk Group	Meat Group	Vegetable & Fruit Group	Bread & Cereal Group

Discussion

This discussion might need to be simplified for some of the children. However, it is vital that they understand the numbers involved, for instance, 3,500 calories equals 1 lb.

Say something like the following:

> The idea of energy balance is crucial to understanding how calories affect your body weight. The energy balance is simply the difference between the number of calories you eat and the number of calories you burn up through exercise and activity.

> If the energy balance is *zero*, your body weight will stay the same. If the energy balance is *positive* (the number of calories eaten is greater than the number of calories burned up), the excess calories will turn into body fat at an approximate rate of 1 lb *gained* for every 3,500 excess calories. Over a period of 1 year, this can add up to a significant weight gain. For example, a positive energy balance of only 150 calories per day (one candy bar!) could add more than *15 pounds* in a year. These numbers actually vary a good deal from one individual to another, depending on the person's level of activity, biology, age, and other factors.

> If the energy balance is *negative* (the number of calories eaten is less than the number of calories burned up), excess body fat will be burned up at the approximate rate of 1 lb *lost* for every 3,500 calories. Over that same period of 1 year, doing an additional 150 calories worth of exercise each day could result in a weight loss of more than 15 pounds.

Group Activity

1. Distribute copies of a calorie-counting book or pamphlet to the group. There should be one copy for each dyad.
2. Start by having everyone look up McDonald's in a brand name calorie counter book. Have them look up the number of calories in the following meal:

Big Mac	541 calories
French Fries	211 calories
Chocolate Shake	363 calories
	1115 calories

Because many of the clients probably need between 1,500 and 2,000 calories per day to maintain their weight, this meal would meet most of their caloric requirements for the entire day, although it would not be nutritionally balanced at all! If they ate much else that day, they would gain weight.

To contrast, have them look up the following well-balanced meal:

3 oz. broiled chicken	165 calories
1/2 cup broccoli w/butter sauce	45 calories
1 slice bread	75 calories
w/1 tsp butter	35 calories
1 medium apple	66 calories
8 oz milk (1% fat)	110 calories
1/2 cup Jello	80 calories
	576 calories

This filling, well-balanced meal contains *half* the calories of the McDonald's meal!

3. Have the clients spend about 5 minutes or so looking up their favorite foods in the calorie-counting book.

Homework

1. As soon as possible, clients are to purchase a good calorie-counting book, if they do not already have one. They should get one with brand names and basic foods.
2. Each evening after supper, parent and child are to sit down together, review their Eating Diaries for the day, and add up their total calories for the day the best they can. The total calories for each day should be written *clearly* in their Eating Diaries (group leaders should check them over next week).

STOPPERS

Leader's Goal: To improve clients' use of stoppers.

Activities: Review of list of stoppers and discussion of experiences.

Discussion

"As was discussed last week, stoppers are things you can do instead of snacking when you get an urge to eat. They should be things that you can start doing quickly and easily and that will make it difficult or impossible for you to eat. Some examples would be to take a walk, chew sugarless gum, or call up a friend."

Group Activity

Ask the people in the group to share some of the 10 to 15 stoppers they were to have brought in this week. You might want to write them on the blackboard. While this is being done, some new ideas will be suggested that some of the clients might want to add to their lists of stoppers. Encourage clients to post their lists of stoppers on their walls and to add new ideas to the list whenever they think of them.

Homework

For next week the clients are to limit their extra snacks to *no more than 4 times* during the entire week. As before, they are to continue recording all extra snacks in their diaries by marking them as *XS*.

MORE STIMULUS CONTROL

Leader's Goal: To help clients make additional use of stimulus-control principles.

Activities: Review of suggestions and discussion.
        Consume food in the eating areas of the home only.

Discussion

"Suppose you have some candy at home. Are you more likely to eat it if it is in a candy dish in the living room or in a box in the top of the cupboard? The point here is that if you have snack foods easily available and visible, you will snack more than if they are out of sight."

Homework

Have clients stop carrying snack foods (except sugarless gum or mints), remove any snack foods from their cars, and remove food from everywhere in their homes except the kitchen and the dining room.
        Do nothing in the eating areas except prepare and eat food.

Discussion

"The first step was to remove the food from near you. The next step is to remove you from the food! If you are in the kitchen doing homework, sewing, reading, or so on, you are much more likely to get hungry and snack than if you are not in the kitchen at all."

Group Activity

Find out from the group what activities they do in the eating areas of their homes besides eat or prepare food. If anyone indicates a problem finding another place for some activity she or he now does in the eating area, help (or better yet, have the group help) her or him come up with alternative ideas.

Homework

Clients are to stop doing anything in the eating areas of their homes except eating and preparing food.

Make eating a "pure" experience.

Discussion

"Has anyone ever had the experience of sitting down in front of the TV set with a box of some snack food and discovering at the end of the program that you had eaten far more than you planned to eat? This happens simply because you are concentrating on something besides your eating and you just don't notice how much you are eating until much later."

Group Activity

Have people share experiences they have had similar to the example above.

Homework

Suggest that clients consider doing *nothing else* (except talking) while they are eating. This includes watching TV, listening to the radio, and reading. Point out to clients that they will enjoy their eating more by focusing on the texture, taste, smell, and other qualities of their food than by concentrating on some other activity.

Summary of Stimulus Control

1. Remove all foods from places other than the eating areas.
2. Do nothing in the eating areas except eat or prepare meals.
3. Do *all* eating, *including unplanned extra snacks*, in the eating areas.
4. Consider doing nothing else while eating, except talking.

EXERCISE

Leader's Goal: To encourage increases in exercise.

Activity: Discussion of how to implement a new weekly goal: 1,000 calories of exercising.

1. This week the goal is to burn up a total of 1,000 calories.
2. If clients were unable to reach their goals last week, be supportive and praise them for what they *did* do, and try to get them to exceed their previous week's total by at least 250 calories.
3. As before, they are to record and graph their exercise both daily and at the end of the week.

Group Activity

Have the parent and the child plan together their exercise for next week and record it on their Weekly Exercise Planning Worksheets.

HOMEWORK ASSIGNMENT

Leader's Goal: To get clients thinking about and working on relevant tasks during the week.

Activities: Provision of information and a handout, discussion of this week's tasks.

1. Parents should review and discuss Handout 4 and what happened in Session 4.
2. Parents and children are to start eating lower calorie foods and to self-monitor calories (every day).
3. Parents and children are to use stoppers, remove all food from noneating areas, eat (but do nothing else except talk) only in eating areas.
4. Participants should agree to continue doing and monitoring exercise (1,000 calorie goal).
5. Parents and children should continue to self-monitor, plan exercise activities, limit the number of meals, and reduce snacking.

NEW CONTRACT

Leader's Goal: To increase compliance.

Activities: Writing and discussion of each client's new contract.

Incorporate nutritional changes (to improve balance in diets) and all elements in the Session-4 homework assignment.

HANDOUT 4:
FOOD, NUTRITION, AND WEIGHT

If you have been following the steps in the first three handouts, you have already begun to make permanent changes in your eating behavior. In the last session, your group discussed stimulus control and exercise. As a result of the first three sessions, the changes you should have made in your eating behavior include:

1. Limiting eating to three meals per day (plus snack for child).
2. Planning when and where you eat.
3. Beginning an exercise program.
4. Becoming more aware of "extra snacks."
5. Taking free food at any time you like.

If you have been doing these tasks, you are making excellent progress. These changes are behind you now. Although we refer to them as tasks, as you repeat them over and over, they will become a part of your behavior and can be performed effortlessly.

It is important to understand that you will probably not have lost very much, if any, weight so far. This is expected. The important thing is that you are on your way to making permanent changes in your eating and exercise patterns. Be assured that weight loss will come slowly at first. More importantly, you are healthier as a result of your exercise program and should notice a feeling of exhilaration and strength from your exercise routine.

In Handout 4, there are several new topics, including (a) balancing your diet, (b) seeing the relationship between calories and weight, (c) using stoppers to reduce extra snacking, and (d) using more stimulus control techniques.

Balancing Your Diet

As we have mentioned, in this program emphasis is placed on good nutrition rather than on a specific list of foods you must eat or avoid. You can lose weight by following the program and continuing to eat your preferred foods. It is hoped that the foods you eat regularly supply you with essential nutrients. This is at the heart of our major recommendation regarding food: Eat a balanced diet!

Let's review just what we mean by a balanced diet. *First,* food is not just calories, but consists of nutrients such as vitamins, minerals, protein, carbohydrates, fat, and important trace elements. We need various amounts of these nutrients to function properly. In fact, the lack of certain nutrients causes improper bodily functioning and can lead to disease. *Second*, some foods provide more essential nutrients than others. Also, there are a few foods, like candy and alcohol, that consist of almost nothing but "empty calories" with little or no nutritional value. Because it is rare for any one type of food to give us all the nutrients we need, we must select a variety to meet our requirements.

Foods are arranged into four groups: milk, meat, vegetable/fruit, and bread/cereal. A balanced diet, then, consists of selections from each of the four groups. It is generally recommended that adults have two or more servings from the milk group per day, which could include milk, yogurt, cheese, or ice cream. Also, you should have two or more servings from the meat group each day. These can be beef, pork, poultry, fish, or eggs. The recommendations for both the vegetable/fruit and bread/cereal groups are four or more servings daily. In addition, you should have a citrus fruit or other source of vitamin C and dark-green or deep-yellow vegetables, as they provide a rich source of essential nutrients. There are a variety of foods in the bread/cereal group such as breakfast cereals, breads, rice, and various noodles. So, in addition to changing your eating habits, pay particular attention to making sure you are receiving a balanced diet. Table 5.1 summarizes these recommendations for children and adults.

Mike P. was a busy high-school honors student who had completed all phases of the program very well. However, his diet was not nutritionally balanced. He rarely ate breakfast, lunch consisted of potato chips and a soda, and for dinner he ate starchy leftovers. He ate few vegetables, and his intake of protein was very low. After reviewing this dietary information, he became more aware of the need for a balanced diet and changed his meals accordingly. In addition to supplying the necessary nutrients, Mike's more balanced diet also helped him lose weight more easily.

Here are some additional dietary tips many people have found helpful in losing weight:

1. Plan your balanced diet around familiar foods.
2. Try not to skip any of your planned meals. This only leads to increased eating the next time you eat.
3. Begin your meal with a salad.
4. Become "calorie conscious" — choose lower calorie foods and methods of preparing foods that do not add to their caloric content.
5. Reduce high-calorie recipes by substituting low-calorie ingredients, without altering their quality.
6. Remember that alcohol has no nutritive value (an 8-oz glass of beer provides 115 calories).
7. Use spices and artificial sweeteners. Six cups of coffee with 2 tsp of sugar per cup adds 216 calories. Artificial sweetener has little, if any, calories.

8. Use artificially sweetened gelatins for desserts and salads.
9. Think of diet soda as a refreshing treat that saves many calories.
10. Go easy on salt. Salt makes your body retain excess fluids.
11. Note that a hot cup of coffee, tea, or bouillon $1/2$ hour before a meal can decrease your appetite.
12. Decrease the caloric intake from butter, oil, grease, and fats by broiling and roasting meats and trimming off the excess fat. By using nonstick sprays and pans, you can cook many foods without adding the extra butter or oil.
13. Try open-faced sandwiches, one-crust pies and cakes without icing.
14. Remember that two slices of thin-sliced bread equal one slice of regular bread.
15. Avoid sugary foods whenever possible. Some research evidence indicates that eating goods high in sugar (most desserts) increases one's craving for more food and more sugar.

Table 5.2 gives some examples of possible switches and their calorie savings. You can think of many others by using a calorie book and looking at what you eat and how it is prepared.

Calories and Weight

Most of you will be surprised to find that it takes fewer calories than you anticipated to maintain your present body weight. With the abundance of food in our country, we consume more than enough to satisfy our body's needs for growth and physical activity.

The idea of an *energy balance* is crucial to understanding how calories affect your body weight. The energy balance is simply the difference between the number of calories you eat and the number of calories you burn up through exercise and activity. If the energy balance is *zero*, your body weight will stay the same.

Table 5.2. Examples of Switches and Calorie Savings

High Calorie	Low Calorie	Calorie Savings
Whole milk (8 oz)—160 cal	Skim milk (8 oz)—90 cal	70 cal
Beer (12 oz)—175 cal	Light beer (12 oz)—95 cal	80 cal
Chocolate cake with icing (2-in. piece)—425 cal	Sponge cake (2-in. piece)—120 cal	305 cal
Butter on toast—170 cal	Apple butter on toast—90 cal	80 cal
Ice Cream (1 cup)—300 cal	Ice Milk (1 cup)—200 cal	100 cal
Duck, roasted (3 oz)—310 cal	Chicken, roasted (3 oz)—160 cal	150 cal
Italian Salad Dressing (1 tbsp)—85 cal	Low calorie Italian Salad Dressing (1 tbsp)—10 cal	75 cal

If the energy balance is *positive* (the number of calories eaten is greater than the number of calories burned up), the excess calories will turn into body fat at an *approximate* rate of 1 lb *gained* for every 3,500 excess calories. Over a period of 1 year, this can add up to a significant weight gain. For example, a positive energy balance of only 150 calories per day (one candy bar!) could add more than several pounds in a year.

If the energy balance is *negative* (the number of calories eaten is less than the number of calories burned up), excess body fat will be burned up at the *approximate* rate of 1 lb *lost* for every 3,500 calories. Over that same period of one year, doing an additional 150 calories worth of exercise each day will result in weight loss. Exercise also helps people lose weight by changing the amount of muscle in the body and other biological processes (*metabolic rate*). So, exercising can help you lose far more weight than suggested by "amount of calories burned up."

Step 1. Keeping Track of Calories. To aid your continuing progress, additional monitoring of your eating is necessary. Although the role of this program is not to put you on a diet, it is important for you to be aware of the caloric content of the foods you eat.

If you do not already own a good calorie-counting book, you will need to purchase one. There are a number of good paperback ones on the market, and you should look for one that includes both brand name foods and basic foods. One excellent book is *Calories and Carbohydrates* by Barbara Kraus (New York: New American Library).

Beginning this week, you and your child are to begin keeping count of your daily caloric intake as accurately as you can. Each night after dinner, the two of you are to sit down together, go through your Eating Diaries, and total up your calories for the day. *Record this daily total in your Eating Diary.* The purpose of this assignment is for you to become much more aware of the caloric values of the foods you eat and to enable you to have an idea of the number of calories you consume in a day. In our next session, we will tell you how you can use this new awareness to gain control over how fast you lose weight.

Step 2. Using Stoppers. In our last session, we asked you to develop a list of from 10 to 15 stoppers, or activities that would interfere with your desire to eat or interrupt ongoing eating. Beginning this week, whenever you are tempted to eat in situations in which you have decided not to eat, you should go over your list of stoppers and engage in one of these activities.

Sometimes you might want to combine two or more stoppers. For example, Ann R., a 9-year-old girl, had included among her list of stoppers (a) chewing sugarless gum, (b) working on her model car, and (c) calling up a friend. She sometimes found that by chewing sugarless gum *and* working on her model car, she would forget about being hungry until her next meal.

As you begin to use stoppers, you will probably find that you want to revise your list. Feel free to do so. In fact, it is a good idea to add new ideas to your list whenever you think of them. This increases the chances that you will find one or more activities that appeal to you whenever you are trying to combat an urge to eat.

It also helps to try to anticipate when troublesome situations are likely to arise and to avoid them. For example, if in the past you have often bought a candy bar while passing a certain vending machine, or you usually buy an ice cream cone whenever you drive by a stand, you might be able to avoid these situations entirely by taking a different route. Taking a different route would reduce the likelihood of having an extra snack. Also, don't forget that you can use free foods as often as you like!

Step 3. Limiting Extra Snacks. For this next week, try to limit eating extra snacks to a total of *no more than 4 times during the entire week.* As before, continue to record extra snacks in your Eating Diaries and mark them *XS.* Remember, though, free foods do *not* count as extra snacks! As an additional help in reducing your tendency to eat extra snacks, we have included a list of ideas that people in some of our previous weight-control groups have found helpful:

1. Remove all visible food from candy dishes, cookie jars, and the like. Make sure that all food in the kitchen is put away and not left on countertops.
2. When storing food in the refrigerator, wrap it in aluminum foil (not plastic wrap) or put it in opaque containers, so it will be less visible.
3. As much as possible do not keep snack foods in the house at all. Those that you do keep, store in the top shelves and behind other groceries, so they are out of sight.
4. Try to buy very few foods that do not require preparation (e.g., sandwich meats, sliced cheeses) because these are easily used for snacking. In general, the more preparation required for a snack, the easier to control impulse eating. If it is necessary to keep sliced meats, cheeses, or whatever for children's lunches, for example, they can be frozen individually on waxed paper and then stored in the freezer without sticking together.
5. If licking beaters or mixing spoons is a problem, before beginning to bake, fill the sink with water and toss the items into the sink immediately after using them.
6. If it is necessary to keep snacks around for other members of the family, try to find snack items that they like but you do not.
7. Before going grocery shopping, prepare a *complete* shopping list. If possible, go grocery shopping no more than once a week. Always go shopping on a full stomach and buy only the items on your shopping list.

More Stimulus Control

To expand your control over various stimuli and situations, you will add three new tasks based on the idea of stimulus control that we introduced in the last session. You are already planning and controlling *when* and *where* you eat each meal.

Now you are going to identify certain areas as food areas. These areas are places where food is stored or eaten and include dining rooms, kitchens, cafeterias, and restaurants.

Step 4. Placing Food in the Food Area. Your first undertaking is to make sure that *all* food in your home is placed in the food area. Ideally, this should be the kitchen. Let's look at some examples. When Beth K. began this step, she found that she had a candy dish in the living room on a coffee table, crackers in the glove compartment of her car, and mints in her purse. Bill P. lived in a boardinghouse and kept pretzels and assorted dips in a nightstand. Beth moved everything to her kitchen, and, because Bill ate his meals in restaurants, he kept this room free of food. All food in your living area, then, should be relegated to a food area. If there is food in any other part of your home or living area, you should place it in the specially designated food area.

Step 5. Discontinuing Noneating Activities in Food Areas. At the same time, non-eating activities should be discontinued in food areas. When you are in the food area, you should be storing food, preparing a meal, or eating. All meals should take place only in the food-storage area. When you are out of the home, the food-storage area might be a cafeteria or a restaurant.

Beth found that she always sewed at the kitchen table. In addition, her children did their homework there, and all the talks over coffee with neighborhood friends took place in the kitchen. To make sure that anyone's presence in the food area was exclusively for meal preparation or eating, Beth moved her sewing machine to the family room, the kids did their homework in their bedrooms, and she found it was more comfortable to serve coffee and tea in the living room than it was in the kitchen.

Step 6. Making Eating a "Pure Experience." Besides storing all food in one area and excluding noneating activities from that area, it it desirable to make eating a "pure experience." By this we mean that it might help if you engage in no activity other than ingesting food while you eat. For instance, do not watch TV, listen to the radio, read the newspaper, or smoke while you are eating. You may converse with family or friends while eating, but do not remain at the table after you finish. While you are eating, try to concentrate as much as possible on the taste, texture, and smell of the food. You will find that you will enjoy eating *more* by eliminating these activities while you eat.

Exercise

Step 7. Increasing Your Exercise. As you know, exercise is a vital part of this program. This week, you are to increase your weekly energy expenditure to *1,000 calories.* Remember, the idea is to be consistent with your exercise program. If, for some unavoidable reason, you miss a planned exercise day, then add more over the next several days to make up for it. However, the routine is what is important and valuable. Watch out! If you do not make this a *regular* part of your life, you will find that excuses come to you easily. By making excuses for not exercising, you are only kidding yourself. As we mentioned in Handout 3, exercise and an active life-style could be the most important and effective inhibitors to extra snacking.

You might wish to vary your exercise, engaging in activities that both stretch and strengthen your muscles and also those that require more energy expenditure, such as jogging, swimming, cycling, and playing tennis. The requirement of 1,000 calories over the next week represents a bare minimum of time that you owe to yourself. It could take you an average of anywhere from 15 minutes to perhaps 30 minutes a day. Remember, however, that you owe this time to yourself. It is one of the most important features of the program for your health, fitness, and feelings of well-being.

Other features that cause some concern for those not accustomed to regular exercise are the feelings of awkwardness and sensitivity to others' impressions. Do not expect to perform these activities with the grace of an athlete who does them every day and has been doing them consistently for years. If you have not exercised, clumsiness is something to expect. However, after several days, you will find that you can perform a number of exercises, including toe touches, jumping jacks, jogging, or swimming, with more ease. It is fun to try more forms of exercise. In addition to you and your child, you might want to try to get the entire family exercising together. Be competitive. They'll love it and you will find yourself getting excited over your progress. Everybody benefits.

If you have ever exercised in public, perhaps you have noticed people looking at you while you are running, walking, playing tennis, or swimming. Individuals who look at you and see you exercising are generally thinking positive and supportive things about your efforts. Perhaps they wish they could be doing the same thing.

Homework

New Tasks This Week

1. Review together what happened at Session 4 as soon as possible after the session is over.
2. Carefully read Handout 4 and encourage your child to read it also.
3. Begin eating a more balanced diet and substituting lower calorie foods for high calorie foods.
4. Every day after dinner, review your Eating Diaries together and figure out how many calories you ate that day. Write down the total calories in your diaries.
5. Limit your extra snacks to *4 times* this week. Continue to record extra snacks in your Eating Diaries and mark *XS*.

6. Use stoppers to reduce extra snacking.
7. Remove all food from the noneating areas of your home.
8. Do nothing in the eating areas but eat, prepare meals, or put away groceries.
9. While eating, do nothing else (no watching TV, reading, etc.) except talk.
10. Continue your exercise program. The goal for next week is an increase of 250 calories burned up (a total of 1,000 calories). Each day record your exercise on your Daily Exercise Records and your Daily Exercise Graphs.
11. At the end of the week, record your total calories burned up on your combined Weekly Exercise Graph.

Continued Tasks

1. Record *all* eating (except free foods) in your Eating Diaries.
2. Eat foods you like and enjoy.
3. Plan together your exercise for next week and record your plans on your Weekly Exercise Planning Worksheets.
4. Plan together your meal schedules for next week and record them on your Meal Schedule sheets.
5. Limit yourself to three meals (plus a snack for the child) per day.

Remember to bring in all materials to the next session!

Chapter 6
Session 5.
Calorie Reductions

REVIEW OF LAST WEEK'S WORK

Leader's Goal: To help reinforce progress and encourage learning of key concepts.

Activities: Dyadic discussions, followed by large-group discussion.
Note the following points, which were covered last week:

1. Continued self-monitoring of eating.
2. Understanding nutrition.
3. Self-monitoring of calories.
4. Limiting extra snacks to four times, recording in Eating Diaries and on Extra Snacks Charts.
5. Using stoppers.
6. Removing food not in eating areas.
7. Doing nothing in food areas that is not food related.
8. Making eating a "pure experience."
9. Exercise, with graphing of results daily and weekly.

Have clients break up into dyads or small groups and identify successful strategies used and problems encountered. Review these in the large group. Point out to clients that there is no expectation that they will have lost weight so far. Some might have lost a few pounds, but some might even have gained a pound or two. The goal so far has been to start building new eating habits; weight loss is a secondary goal at this point in the program.

ESTIMATION OF DAILY
CALORIE REQUIREMENTS

Leader's Goal: To help clients understand why they will need to reduce their caloric intake to lose weight.

Activity: Helping clients to calculate their daily caloric requirements.

1. Multiply estimated "ideal" body weight by a number from 12 to 17, depending on activity level. Problems with this method are that it is difficult to estimate activity level, and it can be very inaccurate, especially if a client is extremely overweight.

2. The actual caloric intake over a 1- or 2-week period, combined with actual weight gain or loss, yields a much more accurate result. For example, if the client ate 35,000 calories during a 2-week period and gained 2 lbs. (7,000 excess calories), the average daily caloric intake for weight maintenance is

$$(35,000 - 7,000) \div 14 = 2,000 \text{ calories per day}$$

The main difficulty with this method is the necessity of very accurate recording of calories. Many clients will have a tendency to underestimate the size of portions or forget "little" things like mayonnaise on their sandwiches. Clients should be encouraged to buy an inexpensive calorie scale if they have difficulty estimating portion sizes. The other problem with this method is that some people have large daily weight fluctuations due to water retention, making it difficult to estimate the actual weight change over a week or two. This problem can be solved by weighing daily for a few days and taking an average.

3. After going over these two methods, help the clients to approximate their daily caloric requirements. Point out that by continuing to self-monitor calories over the next few weeks, they will be able to refine this number and get a much better estimate.

PLANNING OF A LOWER CALORIE
DIET USING EXCHANGE LISTS

Leader's Goal: To help clients decide on an appropriate reduced-calorie plan.

Activities: Review of exchange lists, discussion of appropriate reduced-calorie dietary plans.

1. After clients have come up with an estimate of their daily caloric requirements for weight maintenance, have them figure out the number of calories they would need to eat each day (on the average) to lose weight at a rate of 1 lb per week (reduce 500 calories below maintenance level per day) or $1/2$ lb per week (reduce 250 calories per day). Caloric intakes of less than 1,000 calories are not recommended because of problems achieving a balanced, nutritionally adequate diet at such low levels of intake.

2. *Briefly* explain the idea of an exchange diet list and illustrate how to use the lists at the end of Handout 5. Clients can use the exchange lists to help them plan balanced diets. Note that we are not actually requiring clients to go on a low-calorie diet, but we do want them to become aware of how many calories they can eat if they want to lose weight at a specific rate.

SLOWER EATING

Leader's Goal: To help reduce intake.

Activity: Review of several potentially helpful suggestions.

1. The reason for slowing down eating is to allow fullness messages to get from the stomach to the brain. Normally this takes about 15 to 20 minutes.

2. To slow down eating, clients should place all eating utensils on their plates while chewing each bite. Thus, they should not be cutting the next piece while chewing the previous bite. Also, clients are to cut smaller pieces than they usually do.

3. In the middle of each meal, clients are to *stop eating entirely for 2 minutes.* During this time they can talk, but they are also to concentrate on feelings of fullness before resuming eating.

4. Remind clients that, by eating more deliberately, they will probably find themselves eating less during meals.

5. Encourage talking during meals as a way to help slow down eating.

REWARDS

Leader's Goal: To help clients stay positive toward themselves and recognize the progress they are making.

Activity: Discussion of how to use self-reinforcement concepts.

Review the daily and weekly self-reinforcement concepts discussed in Handout 5. When either the parent or the child meets a daily goal, they should praise themselves for an excellent job. Also, parent and child should praise each other for meeting their goals. This is a part of working together.

LIMITATION ON EXTRA SNACKS

Leader's Goal: To reduce excessive and binge eating.

Activity: Discuss goal: three times per week.

This week the goal is to eat extra snacks no more than *three times* during the entire week.

EXERCISE

Leader's Goal: To increase energy expenditure.

Activity: Planning of the next week's exercise program.

Exercise at the 1,000 calorie level continues for next week. Have clients do their exercise planning during the session.

END OF MEAL SCHEDULING

Leader's Goal: To avoid overtaxing the clients with unnecessary tasks.

Activity: Brief large-group discussion.

It is no longer necessary for clients to formally schedule all of their meals for next week. However, they are to continue eating three meals per day (plus snack for child) and to try to eat at the same place at the same time each day whenever possible.

HOMEWORK ASSIGNMENT

Leader's Goal: To get clients thinking about and working on relevant tasks during the week.

Activities: Provision of information and a handout, discussion of the week's tasks.

1. Have parents review with their children what happened in their session this week and the contents of this handout.
2. Ask parents and children to calculate daily caloric requirements.
3. Encourage participants to use the exchange lists to help plan balanced but calorically restricted diets (aim for $1/2$- to 2-lb weight losses per week for parents, $1/2$ to 1 lb per week for children).
4. Have participants slow down their eating, take time-outs during meals, and reward themselves daily and weekly when they meet their goals.
5. Have participants continue to self-monitor food and exercise (1,000-cal exercise goal) and to use other strategies (e.g., stimulus control, planning, stoppers).

NEW CONTRACT

Leader's Goal: To increase compliance.

Activities: Writing and discussion of each client's new contract.

Include all elements of this session's homework assignments.

HANDOUT 5:
CALORIE REDUCTIONS

As a result of the first four sessions, you should be acquiring more appropriate eating habits. It could be, however, that you are not as yet losing weight. You could be maintaining your weight or even have gained a small amount. There might be several reasons for this. Your food intake at each meal could have increased, you might be building up some muscle tissue, or perhaps you are retaining fluid. Regardless, do not worry! Remember, the objectives of the first part of the program are to establish control over your eating habits and to exercise, with weight loss a secondary goal. If you are following the program, then you are eating systematically and exercising regularly. This is the key to long-term weight loss. So, if you are losing weight, that's fine. If you are developing control of your eating, that's even better.

In this handout, we will be covering several new topics, including (a) estimating daily caloric requirements, (b) using an exchange list for meal planning, (c) chaining, and (d) rewarding yourself.

Estimating Daily Caloric Requirements

There are two basic ways to estimate your daily caloric requirements. The first way is easier and will work reasonably well if you are only moderately overweight (up to 40% over your ideal weight). To maintain your present weight, you must consume between 12 and 17 calories per pound each day, based on your *ideal weight*. If you are very active, your body needs 15 to 17 calories for each pound. if you are inactive, you will require about 12 to 14 calories per pound.

For example, if you are an adult woman, 5′ 4″ tall, with an average build, your approximate ideal weight (without clothes) is 126 pounds (from Session 1). If you are moderately active, you need *approximately* $15 \times 126 = 1{,}890$ calories per day to maintain your weight. If you eat more than this 1,890-calorie level, you could gain weight; if you eat less, you could lose weight.

There are two major problems with this method of estimating daily caloric requirements. One is that it only works if you are moderately overweight. If you are very overweight, this method cannot be used because there are vast individual differences in caloric requirements for very overweight people. The other difficulty with this approach is in estimating your activity level. If you normally get no exercise, work at a desk job, and drive everywhere, it is probably safe to assume that your caloric requirements are near the 12-calorie-per-pound level. Similarly, if you regularly exercise and work as a carpenter, it is probably a good guess that your caloric requirements will be near 17 calories per pound. Unfortunately, few people are at either of these extremes, and it is very difficult to gauge one's activity level accurately.

The second method of estimating your daily caloric requirements is a little more work, but is much more accurate and works for everyone. Last week you began keeping track of your actual caloric intake each day. To compute your current daily requirements, you need to continue to keep track of your actual caloric intake *accurately* for *at least* one more week (preferably longer) and to divide the total number of calories eaten by the number of days, to get a daily average. If your weight stayed the same during this period, the resulting number can be used as an accurate average daily caloric requirement. If, however, you gained or lost weight during this period, you must adjust this figure by 3,500 calories per pound gained or lost as shown in the following example.

Joan A. ate 35,000 calories over a 2-week period and gained 2 lbs. Because a 2-lb gain required eating an excess of 7,000 calories over actual body needs, the estimated daily caloric requirement for Joan to maintain her weight would be calculated as follows:

$$(35,000 - 7,000) \div 14 = 2000 \text{ calories per day}$$

If she wanted to lose weight at a rate of about 1 lb per week, she would need to *reduce* her *average* daily caloric intake to approximately 1,500 calories per day.

In order to use this method, it is very important that you keep *accurate* track of your eating during the baseline period. Common mistakes people make when keeping track of their caloric intake are to underestimate portion sizes and to forget to record "little" things like mayonnaise on their sandwich or cream in their coffee. Unfortunately, these little things add up quickly, and leaving them out will result in an inaccurate estimate of your daily caloric requirements. In fact, unless you are unusually accurate in estimating portion sizes, we strongly recommend buying an inexpensive diet scale and weighing your portions for a few weeks, until you have learned to estimate portion sizes accurately.

Step 1. Compute your Daily Caloric Requirements. If your caloric records over the last week are accurate and complete and you know how much (if any) your weight changed over the last week, use the second method discussed to estimate your daily caloric requirements for weight maintenance.

If your caloric records are not complete, estimate your daily caloric requirements by multiplying your ideal weight by a number from 12 to 17, depending on your activity level. Because this method is not very accurate, it is important for you to begin keeping careful track of your calories so you can obtain a more accurate estimate in the future. In either case, it is important to monitor your caloric intake for at least 2 weeks to get a really accurate estimate of your actual daily caloric needs.

Step 2. Use an Exchange List in Meal Planning. At the end of this handout is some information about using Exchange Lists to help plan balanced, nutritious meals. The Exchange Lists describe foods that are equivalent in calories and in other nutritional dimensions within the four food groups. Use these lists to "mix and match." That is, keep variety in your diet by exchanging one food for another on the same list. These lists might give you some good ideas about the many types of foods you can eat, even in a low-calorie meal plan.

After calculating your daily requirements for weight *maintenance*, decide at what rate you want to try to lose weight and compute the number of calories per day you will have to eat to lose at your desired rate. We do *not* recommend weight loss goals of more than 1 or 2 lbs a week for a parent and $^1/_2$ or 1 lb a week for a child. Remember, you could be more successful in meeting your long-range weight loss goals if you make changes gradually rather than rapidly, as you might have done in the past with "diet" programs.

After you have calculated the caloric intake level necessary to meet your weight-loss goal, use the exchange-list plans to help you plan balanced meals at the caloric level you have chosen.

To illustrate: After Joan A., in the earlier example, calculated her daily maintenance caloric level at 2,000 calories per day, she decided she wanted to try to lose weight at a rate of approximately $3/4$ lb per week. Losing $3/4$ of a pound in a week requires reducing caloric intake by

$$3/4 \times 3500 = 2575$$

calories over the week, or approximately by 400 calories per day. Because her maintenance caloric level was 2,000 calories per day, her new caloric intake level had to be 1,600 calories per day to attain her desired weight-loss goal. To meet this goal, she used the Exchange Plan 1,600 to plan a balanced diet at a 1,600-calorie-per-day level. In general, for most people, caloric goals between 1,000 and 1,500 are safest and most effective, if they also increase their exercise.

Chaining

An important principle you will begin to use in this handout is called *chaining*. It refers to the fact that behavior consists of sequences that can be divided into various components or links. Each link in a chain sets the conditions for the next one to occur. Let's look at eating as a chain. The links in an eating chain might consist of (a) entering the cafeteria or food-storage area, (b) taking a seat, (c) looking at the food, (d) putting food on your plate, (e) picking up eating utensils, (f) cutting the food, (g) putting a bite in your mouth, (h) putting down the eating utensils, (i) chewing, and (j) swallowing. These components are isolated in this example. Rarely do we engage in one link at a time. Rather, we perform several links such as cutting food while chewing, taking a bite while putting food on the plate, and buttering a roll while swallowing. You might even notice that you take a second bite before swallowing the first! This is in addition to talking, listening, or watching TV. In this chaining step, you will accentuate the units of your eating behavior so that it is not an automatic process. By separating the links of the eating chain into distinctive units, you will eat more deliberately and in a more controlled manner.

Step 3. Eat Deliberately. Your task will be to eat in a more deliberate fashion than you have been accustomed to. You should analyze the form that eating takes at each meal and perform one response at a time. If you are eating food that requires cutting, cut a small piece, put your knife down, place the food in your mouth, put the fork down, begin chewing, then swallow. Swallowing sets the occasion for picking up the knife and fork to cut another piece. *Do not* cut another piece while you are chewing. You should be chewing, and the utensils should be on your plate. Apply this deliberate practice to all eating situations and all foods, where practical.

Time Outs

Chaining should at least double the time it takes to eat a meal. This is beneficial, because, as mentioned before, the messages from your stomach about fullness take about 15 to 20 minutes to reach your brain. Slowing down the meal limits the amount of food that you have eaten by the time the fullness message finally reaches your stomach. This gives you advanced warning and helps you avoid overeating.

Step 4. Take a Time-out. To slow down your meals even further, take a *2-minute time-out* from eating in the middle of the meal. There should be no eating during this period. Use this period to concentrate on how full you feel. As you approach the end of your meal, the tendency to eat should be considerably less. If you feel full after the time-out period, stop eating, even if you still have food on your plate. The chaining and time-out tasks will enable you to be more aware of the feelings of hunger as you start to eat and the fullness as you near the end of your meal.

Rewarding Yourself, or Self-Reinforcement

The last major topic of this handout is self-reinforcement, or reward. Briefly, if a behavior is followed by a positive consequence, then the behavior will be increased or maintained in the future. Let's see what we mean by the fact that rewards increase behavior. John B. is a 29-year-old mechanic. Although he works hard, John could not remember doing any "real exercise" since he went to a Boy Scout camp as a teenager. During the second week of this program, John engaged in several exercises at noontime including touching his toes and doing jumping jacks and push-ups. This quickly became a routine. On weekends, his two children joined in. The fact that he was exercising, becoming aware of his body, and doing more active things with his children generated many positive comments from his family, coworkers, and neighbors. The comments, feelings of fitness, and development of control over his life acted as reinforcement for his efforts at exercising. They helped maintain his exercise and enhance his progress in the program. This reinforcement process is a very fundamental law of behavior, and it can be important for your success in the program. It will give you that stick-to-it-iveness.

You are in this program to reap the benefits or reinforcements of weight loss, which include better health and feelings of well-being and attractiveness. However, to reach this long-term goal, you must do the steps as outlined. Rewards will carry you through the program and lock you into permanent change until you finally approach or reach your desired weight.

Certainly, like John, you will be rewarded by others in terms of their comments or glances. They will know that you are on a program to change your life.

However, the rewards that we are talking about now will be administered by yourself and to yourself for your success in the program.

Step 5. Administer a Daily Reward. There are two types of rewards that you can self-administer. The first is a *daily reward*, which consists of the feeling of success or achievement. Each night before you go to bed, review your progress in meeting your weekly contract. Just close your eyes for a moment and think how successful you have been. Think of yourself as shrinking, becoming thinner and thinner, imagine yourself with other thin people at a social group. You fit in. You do not stand out.

It is important that you engage in the rewarding activity of taking a moment out to feel that you are successful in changing your eating behavior. That is precisely what you are doing — making relatively permanent changes in your eating and exercise habits.

The second type of reward is a *weekly reward* and consists of something material or tangible that you like. Tonight then, select an activity or item you would like to use as a weekly reward. This should be something that will act as motivation and help you follow the program closely. In order for you to give yourself this reward, you must achieve all of the goals in your contract for this week. If you earn the reward, you may have it any time during the 3 days that follow the end of the current week. Some weekly rewards might be buying a new record album, seeing a movie, spending special time together with the family, or putting money in a special "bank" for a more expensive reward (like a new coat, a trip, or a bike).

Jessica S., an overweight teenager who liked pretty clothes, chose window-shopping as her weekly reward. If she managed to reach all of her weekly goals, she allowed herself a new scarf, hat, or shirt as an added bonus.

It is important then, that you review, on a daily basis, your weekly contract. You should feel good if you have achieved each goal, and, as you approach the end of the week, you will know whether you will earn your weekly reward.

The reward feature of the program is necessary in order for you to check on your progress and to help lock you into the program. Thus, if you deprive yourself of an activity or thing you really like until you have earned it, this dramatically increases the behavior of adhering to the program. If you decide not to go to the beach on a given weekend unless you have earned the number of points and, if going to the beach is a highly desirable activity, the chance that you will do so is very high.

A couple of words of caution: A reward should *not* be used to keep you from eating extra snacks. This is the function of a stopper. A reward should be what it says — something you have earned by engaging in the tasks of the program. *Remember*, however, if you do not earn a given reward, *you must withhold it until you do*.

Step 6. Limit Extra Snacks. This week your goal is to limit your extra snacks to no more than *three times* during the entire week. Continue to record extra snacks in your Eating Diaries by marking them *XS*.

Step 7. Exercise. This week your goal remains *1,000 calories*. Continue to plan your exercise in advance and to graph it daily and weekly.

Step 8. Discontinue Meal Scheduling. It is no longer necessary for you to schedule your meals in advance for the next week. However, continue to eat three meals a day (plus snack for child) and to try to eat at the same place at the same time each day whenever possible.

Homework

New Tasks This Week

1. Review together what happened at Session 5 as soon as possible after the session is over.
2. Both parent and child are encouraged to read Handout 5 carefully.
3. Calculate your daily caloric requirements to maintain your present weight, using one of the two methods indicated in the handout.
4. Use the exchange lists to help plan a more balanced diet, at a caloric level that will result in weight loss at a rate of $1/2$ to 2 lbs per week (parent) or $1/2$ to 1 lb per week (child).
5. Slow down eating by cutting smaller bites and putting your eating utensils down while chewing.
6. Take a 2-minute time-out in the middle of your meal to lengthen it. Concentrate on the feelings of fullness in your stomach.
7. Reward yourself daily and weekly for keeping your contract.

Continued Tasks

1. Record *all* eating (except free foods) in your Eating Diaries.
2. Eat foods you like and enjoy.
3. Plan together your exercise for next week, and record your plans on your Weekly Exercise Planning Worksheets.
4. At the end of each day, total and record your caloric intakes for the day.
5. Limit your eating to three meals (plus snack for child) each day.
6. Use stoppers to reduce extra snacking. Your goal is no more than *three* extra snacks this week. Continue to record extra snacks in your diaries.
7. Continue your exercise program, plus daily and weekly graphs. This week your goal remains 1,000 calories.
8. Eat only in food areas, do nothing except eat or prepare food in eating areas, and make eating a pure experience.
9. Feel good about yourself and the progress you are making!

Table 6.1. Lean Meat Exchanges

One exchange = 55 calories
(7 grams of protein, 3 grams of fat)

Beef:	Baby Beef (very lean), Chipped Beef, Chuck, Flank Steak Tenderloin, Plate Ribs, Plate Skirt Steak, Round (bottom, top), all cuts Rump, Spare Ribs, Tripe	1 oz
Lamb:	Leg, Rib, Sirloin, Loin (roast and chops), Shank, Shoulder	1 oz
Pork:	Leg (Whole Rump, Center Shank), Smoked Ham (center slices)	1 oz
Veal:	Leg, Loin, Rib, Shank, Shoulder, Cutlets	1 oz
Poultry:	Chicken, Turkey, Cornish Hen, Guinea Hen, Pheasant (all without skin)	1 oz
Fish:	Any fresh or frozen	1 oz
	Canned Salmon, Tuna, Mackerel, Crab and Lobster	1/4 cup
	Clams, Oysters, Scallops, Shrimp	5 or 1 oz
	Sardines, drained	3

Cheeses containing less than 5% butterfat	1 oz
Cottage Cheese, dry and 2% butterfat	1/4 cup
Dried Beans and Peas (omit 1 bread exchange)	1/2 cup

Table 6.2. Milk Exchanges

One exchange = 80 calories
(8 grams of protein, 12 grams of carbohydrate, trace of fat)

Nonfat Fortified Milk

Skim or nonfat milk	1 cup
Powdered (nonfat dry, before adding liquid)	1/3 cup
Canned, evaporated skim milk	1/2 cup
Buttermilk made from skim milk	1 cup
Yogurt made from skim milk (plain, unflavored)	1 cup

Table 6.3. Fruit Exchanges

One exchange = 40 calories
(10 grams of carbohydrate)

Apple	1 small	Mango	1/2 small
Apple Juice	1/3 cup	Melon	
Applesauce (unsweetened)	1/2 cup	Cantaloupe	1/4 small
Apricots, fresh	2 medium	Honeydew	1/8 medium
Apricots, dried	4 halves	Watermelon	1 cup
Banana	1/2 small	Nectarine	1 small

Table 6.3. Fruit Exchanges (continued)

Berries		Orange	1 small
Blackberries	1/2 cup	Orange Juice	1/2 cup
Blueberries	1/2 cup	Papaya	3/4 cup
Raspberries	1/2 cup	Peach	1 medium
Strawberries	3/4 cup	Pear	1 small
Cherries	10 large	Persimmon,	
Cider	1/3 cup	native	1 medium
Dates	2	Pineapple	1/2 cup
Figs, fresh	1	Pineapple Juice	1/3 cup
Figs, dried	1	Plums	2 medium
Grapefruit	1/2	Prunes	2 medium
Grapefruit Juice	1/2 cup	Prune Juice	1/4 cup
Grapes	12	Raisins	2 tbsp
Grape Juice	1/4 cup	Tangerine	1 medium

Cranberries may be used as desired if no sugar is added.

Table 6.4. Bread and Cereal Exchanges (includes starchy vegetables)

One exchange = 70 calories
(15 grams of carbohydrate, 2 grams of protein)

Bread		Cereal		Starchy Vegetables	
White	1 slice	Bran Flakes	1/2 cup	Corn	1/3 cup
(including		Other ready-		Corn on	
French &		to-eat,		Cob	1 small
Italian)		unsweetened		Lima	
Whole Wheat	1 slice	Cereal	3/4 cup	Beans	1/2 cup
Rye or		Puffed cereal	1 cup	Parsnips	2/3 cup
Pumpernickel	1 slice	(unfrosted)		Peas,	
Raisin	1 slice	Cereal	1/2 cup	Green	1/2 cup
Bagel, small	1/2	(cooked)		(canned	
English Muffin	1/2	Grits (cooked)	1/2 cup	or fro-	
Plain roll,		Rice or Barley	1/2 cup	zen)	
Bread	1	(cooked)		Potato,	
Frankfurter		Pasta (cooked)	1/2 cup	White	1 small
Roll	1/2	Spaghetti,		Potato,	
Hamburger		Noodles,		mashed	1/2 cup
Roll	1/2	Macaroni		Pumpkin	3/4 cup
Dried Bread		Popcorn	3 cups	Winter	
Crumbs	3 Tbs.	(popped, no		Squash,	1/2 cup
Tortilla, 6"	1	fat added)		acorn or	
		Cornmeal (dry)	2 tbsp	butternut	
		Flour	2 1/2 tbsp	Yam or	
		Wheat Germ	1/4 cup	Sweet	
				Potato	1/4 cup

Table 6.4. Bread and Cereal Exchanges (includes starchy vegetables) (continued)

Crackers		Dried Beans, Peas, and Lentils	
Arrowroot	3	Beans, Peas, Lentils (dried and cooked)	$1/2$ cup
Graham $2^1/2''$ sq.	2	Baked Beans, no pork (canned)	$1/4$ cup
Matzo $4'' \times 6''$	$1/2$		
Oyster	20		
Pretzels ($3^1/8''$ long $\times$ $1/8''$ dia.)	25		
Rye Wafers $2'' \times 3^1/2''$	3		
Saltines	6		
Soda $2^1/2''$ sq.	4		

Table 6.5. Vegetable Exchanges

One exchange = 25 calories
(5 grams of carbohydrate, 2 grams of protein)

$1/2$ cup of:

Asparagus	Mustard
Bean Sprouts	Spinach
Beets	Turnip
Broccoli	Mushrooms
Brussels Sprouts	Okra
Cabbage	Onions
Carrots	Rhubarb
Cauliflower	Rutabaga
Celery	Sauerkraut
Cucumbers	String Beans, green or yellow
Eggplant	Summer Squash
Green Pepper	Tomatoes
Beets	Tomato Juice
Chards	Turnips
Collards	Vegetable Juice Cocktail
Dandelion	Zucchini
Kale	

The following vegetables may be used as desired:

Chicory	Lettuce
Chinese Cabbage	Parsley
Endive	Radishes
Escarole	Watercress

Starchy vegetables are found in the bread and cereal exchange list.

Chapter 7

Session 6.
Use of Self-Talk and Imagery

REVIEW OF LAST WEEK'S WORK

Leader's Goal: To help reinforce progress.

Activities: Dyadic and small- and large-group discussions.
Discuss:

1. Eating a balanced diet.
2. Slowing down eating, time-outs.
3. Using rewards.
4. Continued self-monitoring of eating.
5. Self-monitoring of calories.
6. Limiting extra snacks and recording them in eating diaries.
7. Using stoppers.
8. Removing food not in food areas and doing nothing except eat and prepare food in food areas.
9. Making eating a pure experience.
10. Exercising with graphing of results daily and weekly.

MORE STIMULUS CONTROL

Leader's Goal: To encourage use of stimulus control principles.

Activity: Brainstorming discussion.

1. The goal is to make the clients' eating area more distinctive, so that eating will become associated with specific cues and will be less likely without them. Examples might be to use special place mats, dishes, napkins, and other items for all meals.

2. Brainstorm with the clients for ideas. Because this is a teamwork effort for parent–child dyads, they might consider getting matching place mats or dishes.
3. To use this technique effectively, clients should try to use their special items whenever they eat, even for snacks.

LIMITED SERVINGS

Leader's Goal: To reduce intake of food by clients.

Activity: Discussion.

Parent and child are to begin limiting their eating during meals to *one serving of each food*. However, they are *not* to increase the size of their servings to compensate. If they are accustomed to eating big meals with multiple servings of favorite foods, this could be difficult for a few days, but assure the clients that their systems will adapt quickly and they will not feel as hungry after a few days.

AVERSIVE IMAGERY

Leader's Goal: To develop a useful technique for inhibiting food intake.

Activities: Modeling and integrating of the group's images of repulsive foods.

1. This is a technique some clients will find useful for reducing urges to eat and others will not, depending on how well they can image.
2. The basic idea is to imagine something very distasteful that will cause loss of appetite. Examples might be imagining yourself becoming nauseous or vomiting or thinking of foods you find repulsive.
3. As a suggested group exercise, have the clients tell you some foods that they strongly dislike. Write these down on the blackboard. Now have the clients imagine as vividly as they can all of these foods mixed together in a big salad bowl. Suggest that they try to picture this scene the next time they have an urge to eat, to try to curb their urge. (Children usually enjoy this activity quite a lot.)

EXCUSES, NEGATIVE THOUGHTS, EXAGGERATIONS

Leader's Goal: To work on problematic cognitions.

Activities: Review and discussion of table in handout.

1. Introduce the idea of negative thoughts and excuses by sharing a few that you have used to avoid exercising or doing some other thing or, alternatively, mention one or two from Table 7.1 (see Handout 6).

2. Have people in the group share some of the negative thoughts, excuses, or exaggerations they have found themselves using during this program and write some of these on the board.
3. Have the *group* come up with positive counterthoughts for the items listed on the board.
4. Stress to the clients that they need to identify the specific negative thoughts that *they* use and to develop specific positive counterthoughts to combat these negative ones. They should then practice saying these positive counterthoughts to themselves, so it will be easier to do when the need arises later on.
5. Have the clients practice for a few minutes during the session.

REDUCED SELF-MONITORING
(PARENTS)

Leader's Goal: To reduce unnecessary tasks.

Activity: Instruction.
   Parents may now reduce their self-monitoring in their diaries to *what, how much, when,* and *where* they eat.

LIMITED EXTRA SNACKS

Leader's Goal: New goal (2 times per week).

Activity: Instruction.
   This week the goal is no more than *2 times* over the entire week.

REWARDS

Leader's Goal: To reinforce progress.

Activities: Review, discussion.
   Clients are to continue to use the daily and weekly reward system. Have parent and child plan together their rewards for next week. Ask if any problems arose with the rewards used last week.

EXERCISE

Leader's Goal: To accelerate weight reduction.

Activities: Discussion, goal setting.
   This week the goal is *increased to 1,250 calories.* Have parent and child do their exercise planning during the session.

HOMEWORK ASSIGNMENT

Leader's Goal: To get clients thinking about and working on relevant tasks during the week.

Activities: Provision of information and a handout, discussion of the week's tasks.

1. Have parents and children review what happened during their groups this week and review this week's handout.
2. Encourage clients to make their eating areas distinctive and to limit servings to one per meal.
3. Have parents reduce their self-monitoring of food to what, how much, when, and where.
4. Encourage the use of aversive imagery and positive counterthoughts.
5. Have clients continue to self-monitor food and exercise (1,250-cal expenditure goal), limit meal frequency (three per day), use stoppers, use stimulus control suggestions, slow down eating, and take time-outs during meals.

NEW CONTRACTS

Leader's Goal: To improve compliance.

Activities: Writing and discussion of each new contract.
Have each person discuss his or her new contract for this week. Keep the goals difficult but realistic.

HANDOUT 6:
USEFUL THOUGHTS AND IMAGES

As a result of the previous sessions, you have begun to make permanent changes in your eating patterns. You now limit your eating to three meals a day (plus snack for a child) with few extra snacks and are making eating a pure experience. You are eating more slowly and appreciating your food more. You are also becoming aware of the food you eat and are planning your eating accordingly. These changes, coupled with increased exercising, will help you to continue to lose weight. They might be becoming a natural part of your life. When these new habits become permanent, keeping your weight down is assured.

New topics for this week include (a) making your eating area distinctive, (b) limiting servings, (c) using aversive imagery, and (d) developing positive thoughts to counteract negative thoughts and excuses.

More Stimulus Control

In the discussion of stimulus control in Handout 3, we noted that people tend to eat in situations that have previously been associated with eating. Strategies for narrowing stimulus control have already been introduced. They include limiting the times and places for eating, making eating a pure experience by not engaging in other activities during meals, and eliminating all noneating behaviors in food storage areas. In this step, you are to extend stimulus control of your eating by making the place in which you eat very distinctive.

In our busy world, people eat in many different places and situations. They often develop the unfortunate pattern of eating just about anywhere. This eating pattern stands in contrast with that for sleeping. Consider the distinctive stimuli associated with your sleeping. You are used to your room, the size and firmness of your bed, and the street or other noises specific to your home. Because your sleeping is under the "control" of these stimuli, you have a difficult time getting a good night's sleep under other conditions. While traveling or visiting, you probably experience a more difficult time sleeping.

Step 1. Making your Eating Area Distinctive. You can learn to limit your eating by making your eating area more distinctive. This can be accomplished in many ways. Distinctive plates, glasses, napkins, tablecloths, or lighting decor are all stimuli that can help make your eating environment more unusual or distinctive. The more of these devices you use, the better. Just remember that the idea is to make your eating area as distinctive for yourself as possible. The following examples will help you think of ways to begin.

Joyce R. decided that she would invest in a bright, red place mat and napkins. Whenever she ate, Joyce always sat at the table with her red place mats and napkins. She also selected a specific place setting, including silverware, china, glasses, and coffee cups, that was different from the others. Whenever she ate, in addition to her place mat and napkins, Joyce ate off her own place setting. Eating at home under these conditions began to influence her eating behavior in several ways. If she wanted to eat, she had to "set the environment" with napkins, china, and place mat. Also, eating under other conditions felt awkward to her as she became accustomed to her new eating conditions.

Ruth and Bob M., a married couple who were in the program together, added a unique and romantic stimulus to their table by always eating with a pair of lit candlesticks. This helped them associate eating with that particular setting and to further limit the occasions for eating. Madeline S., who loved to grow plants and flowers, picked two of her favorite plants to be on her table and join her at all her meals. Other examples include monogrammed dishes, a different color of lighting, and a special chair or position at the table. The more, the better! Be imaginative! Just remember that the goal is to make the place you eat highly distinctive and especially yours.

Step 2. Limiting Servings. Chaining, time-outs, and eating a balanced meal generally help reduce caloric intake. To further decrease your intake, *limit yourself to one serving of each food.* It is important that you not increase your serving size to make up for the reduction in your caloric intake. This reduction might be temporarily difficult if you are accustomed to eating big meals. After several days, however, your body will adapt, and you will notice the reduction in calories.

Aversive Imagery

Aversive images are events or things you avoid or dislike. If they follow an urge to eat, they will usually reduce the tendency to actually eat. Concentrating on these images can help you to overcome urges to eat.

Step 3. Using Aversive Images. Use aversive images as stoppers to help reduce extra snacking. Some examples of aversive images are (a) being forced to eat a food that you hate or that has spoiled, (b) pictures of becoming nauseous or vomiting, (c) a medical article discussing the relationship between heart disease and excess weight, or (d) an unattractive picture of yourself in a bathing suit. These examples are not suitable for everyone, so think of the best ones for you. Feel free to use other images you find personally aversive. When you use mental imagery, you should make the images as vivid and detailed as possible.

Anna T. is a junior executive living in a small apartment who made effective use of aversive stimuli. Over a period of 3 months, she had a total of five extra snacks, which occurred whenever she cleaned her refrigerator. When removing the food while cleaning, she would pick and sample leftover dishes, which would lead to a full-blown eating spree. To overcome this uncontrolled eating, Anna imagined an unfortunate episode that had occurred several years before. While snacking on leftovers, she took several spoonfuls of sour cream before she realized it was spoiled. As a result of eating the sour cream, Anna became very nauseous and vomited repeatedly. Later, when urges for unplanned eating occurred, she simply imagined this event for a few seconds in vivid detail, and her desire to eat quickly decreased.

Thoughts and Your Progress

In this step, we will return to the role that thoughts can play in your behavior. As you will recall, we have discussed the important role a positive attitude about yourself can play in your progress. More specifically, it was recommended in the first session that you abandon any idea of yourself as being basically a fat person. In this step we shall discuss other areas where negative thoughts tend to arise and the destructive role they can play if they are not changed.

Negative thoughts arise in relation to weight loss, progress in the program, exercise, extra snacking, eating habits, and other areas. Each of these areas represents an important integral component of the program, and, therefore, it is important that you not allow negative thoughts to disrupt your progress in any of them.

Perhaps you have noticed that statements you make to yourself often take the form of excuses for not following the program. Our clients report to us that excuses such as "It's too cold to exercise" or "It's a special occasion, I don't have to follow the program" or "Well, I've already blown my diet today, I might as well go hog wild" are very common and often get them in trouble. It will be helpful for you to become familiar with the excuses, negative thoughts, and exaggerations that you use. These thoughts can play a destructive role in keeping you from achieving your weight-loss goal.

Step 4. Developing Positive Thoughts. Table 7.1 illustrates the excuses, negative thoughts, and exaggerations associated with several content areas. For each inappropriate thought, there are listed positive counterthoughts you can use to deal with your nonproductive statements. In general, close examination will reveal that you are merely making excuses, being overly pessimistic, or exaggerating the true nature of the situation. Most people use the same excuses, exaggerations, and negative thoughts over and over, so be prepared! When you hear yourself making these statements, it would help if you were armed and ready with an appropriate positive counterthought. This strategy should make it much easier to stay on the road to your goal.

Let's illustrate several inappropriate thoughts that occurred for Joan Q., a 44-year-old teacher. Early in the program, Joan thought of herself as basically a fat person. If she were to continue with this idea, it would drastically impede her progress, and she would eventually terminate the program. Two weeks into the program, she was able to think of her overweight condition as a result of her eating patterns, unfortunate biology, and inactivity. However, negative thoughts occurred as she experienced difficulties with other areas of the program. For example, after losing approximately 7 lbs by the fourth week of the program, she still felt that she was not making progress. In particular, Joan told herself that "nobody has noticed the 7 pounds I've lost. This just isn't worthwhile, it's just not going to work."

To counter the fact that nobody noticed the 7-lb weight loss on her 175 pound frame, Joan, with considerable practice, was able to say to herself "nobody's noticed the weight I've lost, but certainly I have. I feel better and my clothes are beginning to be a little loose. With 5 to 10 more pounds, people will certainly begin to remark about my accomplishment."

Joan experienced excuses in other areas of the program. In particular, exercise was a problem for her. If it were cold, raining, or she "just didn't feel up to it," excuses were certain to arise. Again, challenging these thoughts took considerable practice on her part. That is, she had to practice positive counterthoughts for those excuses that would interfere with new progress. In fact, it was crucial to her success in the program that she actually practice the counterarguments and anticipate the negative thoughts.

You can expect to have some negative thoughts during the program, particularly when the going gets tough. If you are to be successful, you must be like Joan. It helps to persist like Joan and engage in the three-step process of (a) recognizing the inappropriate statement, (b) labeling it as such and recognizing how it can interfere with your success, and (c) thinking of a counterargument that will serve to motivate you to continue to follow the program closely. Joan started at 175 pounds and, over the course of a year, went to within 7 pounds of her goal of 122. Of course, it wasn't easy. She had lots of arguments with herself along the way.

Patrick R., a 15-year-old high school sophomore, was also troubled by the thought that he was destined to be fat. His father had been overweight and had

Table 7.1. Negative Thoughts and Positive Counterthoughts

Content Area	Negative Thoughts	Positive Counterthoughts
Being overweight and losing weight	I look terrible. I will never be able to lose all this weight.	I've got to begin somewhere. It won't hurt to try. Why don't I just concentrate on losing the first 10 lbs?
	I can never lose enough weight to look decent.	I know other people have been successful in losing weight, so why can't I? I'm losing weight slowly and steadily. Certainly if I keep this up, over the next 6 months I will lose at least 25 lbs more.
	I'm as big as a house.	Who wouldn't be if they ate like me and were as inactive as I am. Besides, houses are built to suit their owners. They can be modified to fit their owners. And that's what I'm doing.
	I've lost 9 lbs and nobody has even noticed.	Well, certainly *I've* noticed the weight loss. I feel better, and my clothes fit better. As I lose more weight, other people are going to notice. I am doing this for myself, anyway.
	It's taking so long to lose weight.	I didn't put it on overnight. I am losing weight gradually and, more importantly, my habits have changed, and I will persist.
Exercise	It's raining, so I'd better not run. I don't want to get my hair wet.	I've run in the rain before, and it can really be fun and enjoyable. It's a little chilly, but, if I wear my rain jacket, it will be okay. Anyway, my hair will dry in a short while.
	I'm too old to exercise.	Exercise makes one feel younger and healthier. If I don't exercise, I'll just grow old faster.
	I've really had a busy day, and I am just wiped out. I don't need to exercise because I burned up a lot of calories running around the office all day.	Well, just think, if I add the calories that I burn up from exercising, it will be just that much more. Also, when I felt like not exercising in the past, when I felt tired and run down, exercising always gave me a lift.
	Oh, I'll do it later.	Later! Gee, I want to go to a movie, so I'd better get it in now, before it's too late. Whenever I've put it off in the past, it never got done.

Table 7.1. Negative Thoughts and Positive Counterthoughts (continued)

Content Area	Negative Thoughts	Positive Counterthoughts
Extra Snacking	Oh, but this is such a special occasion, and I'll only have one.	Well, it might be a special occasion, but then anything can be a special occasion, and I can't start making exceptions. If I have one, it could lead to another and another and another, just like in the past. I've had enough of that.
	It's impossible for me to resist this (e.g., cookie) for they are my favorites.	I'm not on a diet and can eat the things I like. But if I eat this now, it will be an extra snack. Am I really saying that I have no control over what I do—that I have no willpower? I can resist eating anything I want to.
	If I eat (e.g., a brownie), there goes my diet.	If I have an extra snack, it's not the end of the world. But I'd rather not do that.
	I think I'll have one of these. I can go back on the program tomorrow, but now why don't I just live it up and go hog wild.	It's not a matter of going back tomorrow. The real issue is that I don't want to binge, as it might wipe out all the good hard work that I've already accomplished. Besides, I'm no hog!
Eating Habits	Eating like this is awkward. In fact, it's almost stupid.	It sure is nice to *taste* and enjoy food for a change. I didn't know what I was missing when I was shoveling it in.
	What do others think of my eating like this? They must think I'm crazy.	I couldn't care less what others are thinking about me. Besides, I don't look awkward when I eat, just like I'm eating politely and in control of what I'm doing.

died prematurely of a heart attack when he was 55 years old. Pat's uncle was also overweight and suffered from diabetes. Pat did not want to end up like his father and his uncle. This motivated him to lose weight. However, when it was time to increase his exercise and limit his snacking, he would always say to himself "What's the use—no matter what I do, I'm going to be just like my father and uncle." Challenging this negative thought was not very easy for Pat. He countered it with "I am my own person—and can be responsible for myself." After a week of determined effort, in which he doubled his exercise requirement with the aid of a sympathetic physical education teacher, Pat was no longer bothered by the negative thought. He went from 250 lbs to 225 lbs in 12 weeks. Over the summer vacation, Pat lost another 25 lbs and entered college at a much slimmer 200 lbs on a 6′3″ frame.

Step 5. Reducing Self-Monitoring (Parent). Beginning this week, parents may reduce their self-monitoring in their Eating Diaries to recording the same things as their child, namely, what, how much, when, and where they eat.

Step 6. Increasing Exercise. This week your energy expenditure through exercise should be increased to *1,250 calories.* By this time you are well on your way to making exercise and increased activity a regular part of your life, so the small increase should not be overly taxing. Continue to record and graph daily and weekly the calories burned up during exercise. Remember, this is a very important part of your weight-loss program. Weight loss is best achieved by a combination of increasing physical activity and reducing food intake.

Step 7. Rewards. Continue to use the daily and weekly reward system. Remember that it is important to decide on a weekly reward at the beginning of the week.

Homework

New Tasks This Week

1. Review together what happened at Session 6 as soon as possible after the session is over.
2. Read Lesson 6 carefully.
3. Make your eating area distinctive.
4. Limit your servings to one helping of each food per meal—**NO SECONDS!**
5. Reduce recording in your Eating Diary to *what, how much, when,* and *where.*
6. Try using aversive imagery to help reduce extra snacking.
7. Use positive counterthoughts to counteract negative thoughts and excuses.

Continued Tasks

1. Record all eating except free foods.
2. Limit your eating to three meals (plus snack for child) per day.
3. Plan together your exercise for next week and record your plans on your Weekly Exercise Planning Worksheets.
4. Continue your exercise program, plus daily and weekly graphs. This week your goal is *increased to 1,250 calories.*
5. At the end of each day, total and record your caloric intake for the day.
6. Use stoppers to limit extra snacking. Your goal is no more than *two* extra snacks this week. Continue to record extra snacks in your Diaries and on your Extra Snacks Charts.

7. Eat only in food areas, do nothing except eat or prepare food in food areas, and make eating a pure experience.
8. Slow down eating by cutting smaller bites and putting your eating utensils down while chewing.
9. Take a 2-minute time-out in the middle of each meal.
10. Feel good about yourself and the progress you are making!

Chapter 8

Session 7.
Helping Clients
Become Assertive Eaters

REVIEW OF LAST WEEK'S WORK

Leader's Goal: To reinforce progress.

Activities: Dyadic and small- and large-group discussion.
Discuss:

1. Making eating areas distinctive
2. Limiting servings
3. Using aversive imagery
4. Dealing with excuses, negative thoughts, exaggerations
5. Recording calories

See if difficulties with these techniques are noted in dyadic and small-group discussions.

MORE ON SLOWING DOWN EATING

Leader's Goal: To facilitate chaining and reduce intake.

Activities: Instruction, discussion.

1. Clients should be taking a 2-minute time-out during each meal. If they are having trouble remembering to do this, have the group suggest ways to help them remember. Some ideas: having parents and children remind each other, setting a timer to go off in the middle of each meal, and setting aside half of the meal and pausing before eating the second half.

2. To further slow down eating, clients are to pause briefly after each bite in addition to putting down their utensils between bites (which they should already

103

be doing). Each pause should be about *5 seconds long* and should increase awareness of stomach fullness.

GOURMET FOOD APPRECIATION

Leader's Goal: To decrease intake by chaining.

Activities: Instruction, discussion.

To increase their eating pleasure, suggest to the clients that they do the following while eating:

1. Attend to the way the food looks on the plate, noticing its color and consistency.
2. Appreciate the aroma of the different foods.
3. Take small mouthfuls (this will also help slow down eating).
4. Chew the food thoroughly before swallowing.
5. Focus on the taste and texture of each bite.

HOLIDAYS, VACATIONS, AND VISITING FRIENDS

Leader's Goal: To use a planning, problem-solving approach to environmental management.

Activity: Discussion, with examples, of how to plan for coping with problematic circumstances.

1. The focus here is on dealing with changes in the clients' normal daily schedules. Have people in the group share experiences they had that have made it difficult for them to follow the program (e.g., vacations, visiting relatives) and how they tried to deal with these problems. Use the group as a source of ideas as much as possible rather than problem solving yourself.

2. The key point in dealing with changes in normal daily schedules is *planning*. For example, if people are going on a vacation, they need to plan to exercise and plan how they are going to eat well-balanced and low-calorie meals at restaurants or at relatives' homes.

3. A good technique for minimizing problems during holidays or during visits with friends or family is to *educate* the rest of the people involved about the weight-control program *in advance* of the holiday or visit and to ask for their cooperation and help in sticking with it. If the other people are interested, telling them about the program in detail will usually result in their being more supportive.

4. If some of the clients have specific problems when visiting friends or family, and they have not discussed the program with these friends or family, you

might want to give these clients *specific homework assignments* of telling these other people about the program and eliciting their cooperation.

EATING IN SOCIAL SITUATIONS — ASSERTIVENESS TRAINING

Leader's Goal: To develop the social skills needed for weight control.

Activities: Instruction, modeling, role playing.

This topic is a logical continuation of the previous topic in that it focuses on situations where you cannot educate other people in advance (e.g., at a restaurant) or where the other people are not cooperative (e.g., parents or grandparents who equate food with hospitality and love).

1. Introduce the topic with a group discussion of social situations where the clients have had difficulty turning down food. When possible, point out situations that can best be solved by first trying to educate the other people involved and to elicit their cooperation.

2. After the group discussion, talk about the following five key points in assertively refusing food in social situations:

   (a) *Use tone of voice* and *facial expression* to convey a sincere and *firm* conviction.

   (b) Maintain *eye contact* while speaking.

   (c) *State clearly* desires and interests.

   (d) *Compliment the host or hostess* on preparation of food and other achievements in conjunction with a refusal.

   (e) *Suggest an alternative* such as tea or coffee instead of alcohol, a fruit or vegetable instead of dessert, taking leftovers home instead of having seconds, and so on. This allows the host or hostess to feel satisfied that he or she is doing a good job.

3. Have the co-leaders role-play an assertive food-refusal situation as a model for the group. If possible, have someone in the group provide a real situation for the role play.

4. Try to get some of the clients to role-play dealing with a problem situation for them, so they can receive feedback from the group. Try to get the children involved in doing the role plays. For example, if a parent has problems refusing food when visiting his or her parents, you might have the child play the part of the grandparent who is trying to push food on the parent.

EXERCISE

Leader's Goal: To accelerate weight reduction.

Activity: Goal setting (to 1,500 calories per week).

This week the goal is *increased to 1,500 calories.*

HOMEWORK ASSIGNMENT

Leader's Goal: To get clients thinking about and working on relevant tasks during the week.

Activities: Provision of information and a handout, discussion of the week's activities.

1. Have parents and children review and discuss Session 7 and Handout 7.
2. Ask parents and children to continue to use chaining principles by pausing after each bite and attending to all sensory aspects of eating (i.e., gourmet eating).
3. Encourage participants to manage their food-related environments by planning for alterations in daily routine and by practicing and being assertive (food refusal).
4. Have clients streamline their self-monitoring of food further to include only what, when, and how much.
5. Encourage participants to continue with all other aspects of the program (e.g., exercising to 1,500-cal expenditure).

NEW CONTRACTS

Leader's Goal: To improve compliance.

Activities: Writing and discussion of clients' new contract.
Have clients write and then discuss their new contracts.

HANDOUT 7: BECOMING
AN ASSERTIVE EATER

Most of the steps that follow this week are extensions of those presented in the first 6 weeks. It is important that you have the initial steps down pat. Mastery of 1 week's tasks is a must if you are to be successful with the next. Moving ahead too quickly usually causes problems. Take your time and be persistent; chip away at your problem areas. You will get there. Whenever you encounter problems in following the program, always refer to past sessions to find out how to deal with them. Remember, if, for some reason, you should stray from the program, recognize it as a temporary break and return to the recordings, assignments, and other tasks immediately.

Time-outs and Chaining

If you have had trouble remembering to take a 2-minute break in the middle of each meal, then you might want to devise something that can serve as a reminder. One way would be for the person with whom you eat to remind you.

A more extreme and certain method is to make a note to yourself, roll it in a rubber band, and put it on the wrist of your dominant hand. Movements of this hand (particularly those involved in eating) will bring the message into eye contact and be a constant reminder of the time-out task. Other helpful methods are to set the kitchen timer or an alarm watch to go off somewhere in the middle of the meal or to set aside half of your food before you eat it and stop when you finish the first half. For example, if you are eating a sandwich, cut it in half, stop for your time-out after you have eaten the first half, then continue if you are still hungry.

Step 1. Pausing While Eating. In order to further lengthen the chain of eating behaviors, this week begin to *pause briefly after each bite*. Each pause should be approximately *5 seconds* in length and should enhance your awareness of stomach fullness.

Food Appreciation

The purpose of this program is not to deprive you of your eating pleasures but to increase these pleasures. In conjunction with decreasing the amount of food you eat, you should also begin to eat like a gourmet, by enjoying your food to the fullest with all of your senses — its sight, smell, texture, and taste.

Step 2. Increasing your eating pleasure. You will find that the following procedures will help you to increase the pleasure of eating:

1. Attend to the way your food looks on the plate, noticing its color, consistency, and other qualities. Try to serve your food in a pleasing manner (don't just grab a bologna sandwich).
2. Appreciate the aroma of different food items.
3. Take small mouthfuls (this will also help you to lengthen your chain of eating behavior).
4. Chew the food thoroughly before swallowing.
5. Notice the texture of each bite.
6. Savor the taste of each bite.

By following the above procedure, you should find that you enjoy eating more than you did before you began this program, even though you are eating less!

Alterations in Your Environment

At this point, it would be helpful to discuss a problem area that might lie in the path of your progress. Most people have a daily schedule or routine that includes both work and leisure activities. In the last few weeks, focusing on the program and its steps should have become a natural part of your daily routine.

However, what happens when your schedule is disrupted? All of us have visitors, take vacations, become sick, or take on extra work loads. Sometimes these events are unanticipated, and suddenly we are in a new situation.

Step 3. "Hanging In". At times you might feel like letting the program take a back seat. Do not let this happen! Like a Boy Scout, you must be prepared. Your life and happiness are at stake. Disruptions in your schedules do not have to involve abandoning or dramatically altering the program. If you are ill, you might not be able to exercise, but you can certainly adhere to your limitations regarding eating. Also, exercise and changes in eating can be incorporated into any vacation or travel.

Anna T. is a busy, middle-aged executive who had no trouble sticking to the exercise and eating components of the program while keeping a strenuous schedule. During the week of this seventh session, she had an extended bout with the flu, which kept her at home. She was not able to exercise for 4 days during this period. However, she used this time to become more aware of the role food played in her life. She spent her convalescence thinking about her program and how she could improve it.

Another important problem, typical for many people, was found by Sally F., who lives alone in a small apartment. She was progressing through the program very well. However, she found that occasional visits with her family in another city were extremely difficult. Her mother equated a hearty welcome with rich pastries. Sally's father took the entire family out to eat at a restaurant where the food was served family style and second helpings were encouraged. Sally was confronted with a very difficult choice. She did not want to discontinue visiting her family. What could she do? She decided to enlist her family's aid and to educate them about her program.

At first, her parents challenged her. She heard that she was not "that overweight" and that when she had been thin, years ago, she had looked frail, weak, and sickly. Her mother remarked "You'll never stay on that diet program." Yet Sally was persistent. She informed her parents of her determination to lose weight and of the fact that the program had helped her a great deal. She was able to reason with them and explain the nature of the program. By showing that she wanted to be "in control of her eating" and practicing strict eating management she was able to handle both the visit and staying within the program extremely well. On subsequent visits to her parents, activities associated with eating decreased, with everyone making a conscientious effort to help Sally instead of hinder her.

It is important to be ready to cope with both unscheduled or scheduled alterations in your daily routine. Managing your environment and the circumstances under which you eat and exercise may be difficult at times, but, as with Anna and Sally, it is not impossible.

Eating in the Presence of Others

There are many situations in the course of your daily routine that increase the tendency to eat. You can avoid many of these circumstances, but often it would be difficult or socially awkward to do so. For instance, we all attend celebrations, parties, and feasts and have parents and friends who occasionally fix our favorite meal. You can apply previously learned strategies to social situations and therefore participate in social activities without allowing eating to be the focus of your enjoyment. You are not at a social activity just to eat, but also to enjoy the company of others.

Planning your mealtimes wisely can help you participate actively in many special occasions. Ruth and Bob M. were often faced with conflicts caused by their busy social schedule. Bob is an executive, and his presence at social functions was expected. Instead of being forced to stay home or not eat the food at weekend cocktail parties, Ruth and Bob planned their meal schedule to anticipate extra eating. On the day of a party, they would eat a late breakfast and then lunch at 2 or 3 o'clock. This would make it possible to wait until 7 or 8 o'clock for the evening meal. They would eat the food served at a party or other social gathering as their third meal, rather than as an extra snack.

In many situations it is common for party givers or family members to insist on your eating more than you had planned. They see this as a way of insuring that you enjoy yourself. Perhaps you have often heard such statements as "I made it just for you," or "Oh please, at least try one" or "This is no time to be on a diet." These statements are surely difficult to resist, particularly when the food is so attractively prepared. Yet all is not lost, for there is something you can do.

Step 4. Asserting Yourself in Food-related Situations. We have found that being able to assert your needs and desires in social situations is an excellent alternative to being forced to eat. This probably sounds like something that is easier said than done. However, as you apply the ideas outlined in this section, you will realize that being assertive in food-related situations is a skill that, with some practice, you can easily use.

You might be able to speak up for your rights in a variety of settings. But, when offered food by a friend or by your parents, you might not be assertive enough to say no. This is not uncommon. Even the most assertive individuals have a difficult time expressing themselves properly when it comes to food. There are many examples of lack of assertiveness in food-related situations. Several of the most common include being forced by a persistent hostess or host into accepting leftover hors d'oeuvres at a party, being unable to request that restaurant food be cooked to your low-calorie specifications, and failing to pass up unwanted second portions for fear of offending your hostess or host or your parents.

Let's look at several specific examples of difficulties with assertiveness in food situations. After starting the program, Jane L., a 13-year-old girl, did not want to attend parties because she was afraid that she would snack too much. She said that she could never lose weight and attend parties at the same time. The conflict between maintaining her active social life and losing weight was a difficult problem. Jane did not want to give up either her social life or her desire to lose weight. She recognized that reducing her social activities would be an instance of the *overweight paradox*. That is, Jane knew that, if she found herself staying home more often with nothing to do, she would be more likely to have extra snacks. She might have ended up adding even more to her 160 lbs. At this point in the program, Jane had begun to lose weight at a comfortable $1/2$ to 1 lb a week. We decided then to focus on teaching her to change her behavior in these social situations rather than avoid them. The first step in working with Jane was to analyze exactly what was going on in these situations. She reported frequently hearing statements such as "Try one, they are so good," "I'll be so upset if you don't take one of these." What made matters worse was that many of these individuals were mothers of Jane's close friends or of Jane's relatives.

Ruth L., a 20-year-old college student, had a similar problem, which revolved around her family. Whenever she visited her parents, she always ended up eating more than she had planned. In fact, Ruth's mother insisted on second helpings and responded to Ruth's protests with hurt feelings. Ruth's mother would either feel that she didn't enjoy the food, that something was wrong and perhaps Ruth was sick, or that Ruth was, in fact, mad at her.

A third example is the case of Susan R., a 23-year-old keypunch operator. She had a slightly different problem. Susan was enrolled in a YWCA swimming class 3 nights a week with a group of friends. Because the class was from 5:30 to 6:30, Susan and her friends would postpone eating until after the class, at which time they would all go to a local restaurant. Susan had every desire to eat foods that would be appropriate to her weight-loss efforts. However, most of the foods on the menu were prepared with a considerable amount of butter and grease and were often covered with rich sauces. She had considered requesting that her food be prepared without grease and sauces, but feared causing a big scene with the waiter. Consequently, Susan often found herself forced into eating inappropriately when she went out.

Before we discuss how these individuals solved their difficulties with being assertive, let's look at the various components of a good assertive response in food-related situations. These are (a) a firm tone of voice, (b) eye contact, (c) desires stated in a clear and unambiguous fashion, (d) compliments to the host or hostess, and (e) suggested alternatives. Each component is important in a good food-refusal response. So, let's look at them in more detail.

First, your *tone of voice* and *facial expression* must show that you are serious about your needs. Specifically, your voice should not waver, and your expressions should not lead your hostess or host to believe that there is some doubt in your own mind as to your desires. This will only lead to continued pushing of food at you.

Second, *eye contact* is extremely important. If you don't look the other person in the eyes, that person will believe that you are not sincere about what you are saying. So, look straight at your host or hostess when you express your desires.

Third, your desires and interests must be *stated clearly*. If you wish to refuse food, don't say "I don't think I want one" but say, "No, thank you!" Being tentative about whether you want food or not merely leaves doubt in your hostess or host's mind as to your real intentions. Similarly, if a waiter or waitress hears "if it's not too much bother, could you . . . " he or she is likely to underestimate the importance of your request and tell you that he or she cannot accommodate you. So, state clearly what you want the waiter or waitress to do, for instance, "I would like you to . . . " or, "This is not the way I asked you to prepare this, so please take it back." These responses are much more definite and signal the waiter or waitress regarding the importance of your request.

These components will be important for you to keep in mind in any food-related assertion situation. Two other components will be particularly important in social situations where you must deal with hosts or hostesses who are anxious to make sure that all their guests are enjoying themselves.

One of the most effective things that you can do is to *compliment the hostess or host of a party or your parents on the preparation of their food*. This fourth component is particularly helpful if you are worried that your failure to sample the food might offend your hostess or host and be taken as a sign that you are not enjoying yourself. The compliment should consist of a statement describing the attractiveness of the food and its taste or smell. Additionally, you might wish to remark to your hostess or host that you are having a good time. This makes her or him aware of the good time you are having and is often sufficient to halt their worrying about getting you to eat.

The fifth component of a good assertive response is *suggesting an alternative*. As you will recognize, many hosts and hostesses, and particularly parents, are not satisfied until they have given you something or until they feel that you are satisfied in every possible way. So, in addition to the four previous components, it is also helpful to suggest an alternative to what your hosts or parents are offering. This can simply be done by asking for a cup of tea, coffee, or other low-calorie drink. In addition, you might avoid eating high-calorie foods such as rich pastries or desserts by requesting an alternate low-calorie food such as a fresh vegetable or a fruit. Another option is to suggest that you would enjoy having the food offered at a later time, such as with your next meal or for lunch the following day.

Well, let's see how Jane, Ruth, and Susan handled their difficulties. After some practice, Jane was able to look her hostess or host directly in the eye and respond in a rather firm, sincere, and direct fashion similar to the following:"No, thank you. I really am serious about not eating any more. This is a great party, and I am having a fun time. Oh! I would appreciate having a glass of water. Thanks a lot!" We can see that Jane (a) was direct and straightforward in her tone of voice, (b) made strong eye contact, (c) stated her position very clearly, (d) complimented her hostess or host, and (e) suggested an alternative.

The same success was achieved by Ruth in her difficulties with her mother. She was able to (a) look at her, (b) say in a firm and sincere manner (c) "Mom, no thank you. I just couldn't take a second helping. (d) The food was great, and I'm really full. It was delicious. It's great to be home and a pleasure eating your good home-cooking. You work so hard to make everything just perfect. (e) I would like to have some of the casserole if any is left over. I'd love it for lunch tomorrow."

Susan, you will remember, had difficulty eating out because of her inability to request that foods be prepared in a low-calorie manner. After practice, Susan was able to express herself in a manner similar to Jane and Ruth's. She would order a meal by saying "It is very important that my food be cooked the way I request it. I would like plain broiled chicken with no sauce and plain boiled vegetables without any butter. Will that be possible?" (It will not be possible to get everything you want in every restaurant. Sometimes you might have to choose a different item, which can be prepared in an appropriate manner.) She stated her requirements and requested appropriate information from the waitress or waiter. If the food is prepared differently from the way she requested, Susan has her full right to express her dissatisfaction and ask that it be returned.

Now, you should review your eating behavior in social situations. You might refer to the observations of your eating, or just think of how things are when you are enjoying the company of others and food is present. Do you experience any difficulties in refusing food in these situations? Can you resist the offers or demands of others? Do you ever find yourself eating food that you did not really want?

To insure that you are capable of being assertive in food-related situations, we suggest that you practice the appropriate food-refusal responses for the situations that usually confront you or that could confront you in the future. Practice is necessary for you to learn how to be appropriately assertive.

How do you think Jane, Ruth, and Susan were able to be assertive and refuse food? It certainly didn't come naturally; it was a problem for each of them. The key is practice, and, like everything else, practice makes perfect in being assertive. To aid your practice, we suggest that you use the following rehearsal strategy:

1. Consider the situations in which it has been difficult for you to assert yourself concerning appropriate eating.
2. Prepare an appropriate food-refusal response for each of these situations. Keep in mind the five important components we discussed: (a) be sincere, (b) maintain eye contact, (c) clearly state your desires and interests, (d) compliment your host or hostess, and (e) suggest an alternative.

3. Practice these responses in a mirror. Make sure that you have included all the appropriate components. That is, look yourself directly in the eyes, state your response clearly with a firm sense of conviction, imagine that the hostess or host persists, state your compliments, and suggest an alternative.
4. Role-play the same situation with a friend after you have practiced in this solo fashion. Role playing is simply acting out a situation as it might happen. Inform the friend of exactly what he or she is to do, describe the scene, then you and your friend role-play. It is helpful for your friend to be a little pushy, just as the troublesome host or hostess or parent might be.
5. Ask your friend for feedback on how well you performed after you have role-played the situation.

After several simulated role plays for each troublesome situation, you are ready to handle the problem situation or any new ones that might occur. Each time you assert your right not to eat unwanted food, it will become easier and easier, and you will feel better and better.

At times, even the most persistent attempts to refuse food will not be accepted. After you have tried all of the strategies previously outlined, including asking your hostess or host for a permissible noncaloric substitute or telling her or him that you will be glad to take some leftovers home to eat when you are hungry (at your next meal), you might need to leave the situation if your approach did not work. This could include going to talk to someone else at a party, stepping outside for fresh air, or going home early if necessary.

Step 5. Reducing Self-Monitoring. Beginning this week, both you and your child can reduce your self-monitoring of *scheduled* meals to *what* and *how much*. However, for any extra snacks, continue to record *when* and *where* you ate the snack, because this could reveal patterns that need further work to change or eliminate them. As before, continue to total your calories each night and record the total in your Eating Diaries.

Step 6. Increasing Exercise. This week your exercise goal is to burn up *1,500 calories*. Continue to record and graph daily and weekly the number of calories burned up during exercise.

Step 7. Using the Reward System. Continue to use the daily and weekly reward. Remember, it is important to decide on weekly rewards in advance. You should also begin to plan other more extensive and elaborate rewards. Give yourself larger rewards for staying with the program for a month. Examples might be buying a new dress or a bathing suit, spending a weekend in the country, or purchasing a new tennis racket. You might decide not to take one of these elaborate rewards until you have gained your weekly reward for four consecutive weeks.

Homework

New Tasks This Week

1. Review together what happened at Session 7 as soon as possible after the session is over.
2. Read Handout 7 carefully.
3. Further slow down your eating by pausing after each bite.
4. Begin to increase your appreciation of food by eating like a gourmet.
5. Anticipate changes in your daily schedule and make plans to handle it.
6. Don't let others control your eating — be assertive!
7. Reduce routine self-monitoring to *what, when,* and *how much* you ate at each meal. For extra snacks, continue to mark XS.

Continued Tasks

1. Record all eating except free foods. At the end of each day, total and record your caloric intake.
2. Limit your eating to three meals (plus snack for a child) each day.
3. Plan together your exercise for next week and record your plans on your Weekly Exercise Planning Worksheets. This week your exercise goal is *increased to 1,500 calories.* Continue to record and graph your exercise as before.
4. Use stoppers to limit extra snacks. Your goal remains at no more than *two* extra snacks this week. Continue to record extra snacks as before.
5. Maintain good stimulus control: all food and eating only in food areas, eating as a pure experience, a distinctive eating area.
6. Slow down eating and take a 2-minute time-out in the middle of each meal.
7. Continue your daily and weekly rewards. Consider adding a larger monthly reward.
8. Feel good about yourself and the progress you are making!

Chapter 9

Session 8.
Non-eating Alternatives
for Coping with Stress

REVIEW OF LAST WEEK'S WORK

Leader's Goal: To reinforce progress.

Activities: Dyadic and small- and large-group discussion.
Briefly discuss:

1. Slowing down eating
2. Appreciation of gourmet food
3. Dealing with holidays, visiting friends, and so forth
4. Assertiveness training

Ask dyads or small groups to focus on how well they used techniques this week. Work on problems in the larger group.

MAINTENANCE OF WEIGHT LOSS

Leader's Goal: To orient clients to what they need to do for long-term success.

Activities: Instruction, discussion.
1. Review the five factors discussed in Handout 8 relating to postprogram weight-loss maintenance:
   (a) Coping with stress.
   (b) Trait thinking.
   (c) Continued self-monitoring.
   (d) Continued exercise.
   (e) Continued social support.

RELAXATION

Leader's Goal: To teach a useful coping skill.

Activities: Relaxation training, discussion.

1. Assess how big a role stress currently plays in eating for people in the group and how much of a role it has played in the past. You might also want to talk about the effects of stress and anxiety on people in other settings. Use this as a lead-in to the relaxation training.
2. Do a relaxation-training session with the group (follow the Handout 8 section on relaxation).
3. Review people's reactions afterward.
4. Ask clients to try it themselves a few times over the next week, even if they currently do not feel that they have a stress-related problem.

EXERCISE

Leader's Goal: To accelerate weight reduction.

Activities: Goal setting, discussion.
Continue exercise at the 1,500-calorie level again this week.

HOMEWORK ASSIGNMENT

Leader's Goal: To get clients thinking about and working on relevant tasks during the week.

Activities: Provision of information with a handout, discussion of the week's tasks.

1. Have parents and children review and discuss Session 8 and Handout 8.
2. Encourage parents and children to practice the relaxation procedures presented in this handout.
3. Ask parents and children to continue all aspects of the program (exercise goal is now 1,500 cals).

BEHAVIORAL CONTRACTS

Leader's Goal: To improve compliance.

Activities: Goal setting, discussion.
Include practice with relaxation in this week's contracts.

HANDOUT 8:
COPING WITH STRESS

By this point in the program you have mastered most of the specific steps necessary to change your eating behavior permanently. You should now be losing weight at a steady rate. The remaining steps in this program are concerned primarily with learning how to continue this steady weight loss and how to deal with problems that could arise in the future.

Maintaining Weight Loss

A large amount of research has been done on maintaining weight loss. Five factors that seem to be important are (a) coping with stress, (b) overcoming "trait thinking," (c) continuing to self-monitor, (d) continuing to exercise, and (e) continuing to get support from other people.

Coping with Stress. For many people who fail to maintain weight loss, the first major eating crisis or binge occurs during a highly stressful time. It is very common for people to eat more during times of stress, and it is very important for you to realize that eating is a specific reaction to the stressful situation. Such a binge is *not* an indication that you have failed and should not be used to justify giving up the effort to lose weight. Later in this handout we will be describing one way in which you can directly reduce the effects of stress. In any case, you should realize that an occasional setback is common and should be viewed as only a *temporary* problem. The problem does not show that you are incapable of losing weight.

Overcoming "Trait Thinking". Research evidence indicates that many people who are overweight, smoke, or have other problems that are difficult to overcome think of their problems as permanent personality traits. For example, they might think of themselves as being fat in the same way as they think of themselves as being tall or dark-haired. There is a problem with this style of "trait thinking." It increases the tendency to view any problem (e.g., overeating under stress) as confirming this permanent view of themselves as being fat rather than to view the problem as a temporary setback. In other words, people who use trait thinking blame themselves for the problem. It would be better to blame the problem on the specific situation that triggered it.

Continuing to Self-Monitor. It is very desirable to continue to self-monitor your eating on a permanent basis. Ideally, you should continue recording what and how much you eat, as well as the calories, but at least just keeping track of your caloric intake will allow you to tell how well you are doing. This will make it easier for you to realize if you are beginning to develop problem areas that need to be attacked more vigorously. Another reason for continuing to self-monitor your eating is that it keeps you focused on maintaining the eating habits and eating environment you have developed by following this program. Remember, the changes you have made in your eating must be maintained in order for you to continue to be successful in controlling your weight.

In addition to continuing to monitor your eating on a daily basis, you should monitor and record your weight on a regular and permanent basis. The best way to do this is to put a weight chart on your bathroom wall near the scale and record your weight on a weekly (or biweekly) basis. You should plan to do this *permanently*. Make it as much a part of your life as brushing your teeth! If your weight drifts upward by a few pounds after you have reached your goal weight, then you'll know that you need to get to work again.

Self-monitoring is a very important component in successfully maintaining control over your weight. Research has shown that people who continue to self-monitor are much less likely to return to old problematic habits than people who stop self-monitoring.

Continuing to Exercise. Aside from the many major health-related reasons for maintaining a regular exercise program, follow-up studies on people who have been in weight-loss programs similar to this one clearly show that those people who continue to exercise on a regular basis do better in continuing to lose weight or maintaining weight loss than those people who stop exercising. As we have repeatedly stressed, exercise is a very important component of a successful weight-loss program.

Continuing to Get Support from Other People. Several research studies have found that people in this type of weight-loss program are more successful in continuing to lose weight if they continue to receive support from important people in their lives. It is important for parents and children to continue to give each other support and encouragement about your eating and exercising behaviors.

Using Relaxation to Cope
with Stress and Curb Impulse Eating

It is generally true that uncontrolled eating and snacking is well controlled after 4 weeks on this program. Participants use a variety of techniques such as stoppers, and they become accustomed to eating only three meals a day. If extra snacking does occur, it is most likely related to some emotional state. To deal with this effectively, we should first assess under what conditions it occurs and then plan an effective strategy to control it. To determine whether your snacking or uncontrolled eating is related to an emotional state, refer to your Eating Diary. Are there times when you eat that you describe yourself as feeling angry, bored, anxious, or just upset? In these situations, you might not be in control of your eating because some event or thought leads to an emotional reaction, which leads to eating or snacking.

Let's take the example of Sam R., who was a dispatcher of service trucks for a large appliance firm. His job was full of stress and tension, particularly in the morning, when trucks were on the road and calls came from other customers seeking assistance. Sam's job entailed assigning the service people to customers, estimating the duration of a job, and informing customers of when they could expect service. Additionally, some service calls needed to be scheduled for priority service, stoves and refrigerators ranking far ahead of washing machines, trash compactors, and ovens.

Sam began his day at 7:30 a.m. and had lunch at 11:30 a.m. Lunch was more of an escape from the demands of the job than a time in which he could enjoy a meal. In fact, Sam ate a small amount during lunch, primarily because he was still overcome by the tension and stress of his hectic morning.

Sam's difficulties increased shortly after lunch, when he would be confronted by his supervisor with a number of complaints from customers who demanded immediate service. From approximately 1:00 p.m. to 3:30 p.m., Sam was so upset that he ate continuously. While he sat at his desk talking with customers on the phone and service people in the field, other workers supplied him with an assortment of hamburgers, french fries, pies, and cookies from vending machines. It was obvious that Sam would have to make some major changes at work in order to lose weight.

In the initial phases of the program, Sam tried using stoppers to limit his after-lunch binges. This did not work. It became clear that he would have to directly attack the tension and stress that led to his overeating. We trained Sam to use a relaxation procedure that was very effective.

A very important part of the relaxation technique is that it must be practiced several times a day in a comfortable environment before it will help in a stressful environment. At first, Sam practiced the relaxation technique at home in a comfortable setting. On working days, he practiced the technique 2 to 3 times during the evenings in the comfort of his own home and up to 6 times over the weekends. He did this for approximately 1 week prior to using it in the more stressful work environment.

Sam used the following procedure, which you are encouraged to use if you find that some of your snacking is related to being anxious, nervous, or otherwise emotionally upset. The relaxation training consists of a sequence of exercises that alternate between tensing muscle groups and relaxing them. By first tensing a muscle, it is much easier to "let it go" and relax it. With your muscles becoming more and more relaxed, it is easy for you to calm down and be in control of your behavior.

You should sit in a comfortable chair in a quiet room with low light. Close your eyes and then focus your attention on various muscle groups, alternating tension and relaxation. Settle back in the chair, take a deep breath, let it out slowly, close your eyes and make your mind a complete blank. Extend your arms directly in front of you, clench your fists, and tighten all the muscles in your arms. Hold this for 5 seconds, then say "Relax," as you let your arms slide to the arms of the chair and relax. Focus on the immediate contrast between the tension that was in your arms and the developing relaxation. Let your arms and hands relax for 30 to 60 seconds. During this time, you should notice the relaxation spreading and how your hands and arms feel noticeably different from the rest of your body. Repeat this procedure for a second time, tensing for 5 seconds and relaxing for 30 to 60 seconds.

Follow the same procedure for other muscle groups. *Face*—squint your eyes, crease your forehead, and clench your teeth together. Hold the tension for 5 seconds, then "Relax." Notice the relaxation spreading over your face. Keep relaxing for 30 to 60 seconds. Repeat the procedure. *Upper trunk*—take a deep breath, shrug your shoulders, tense the muscles in your chest, neck, and back. Hold the tension for 5 seconds, then "Relax." Notice the relaxation spreading over your upper trunk. Keep relaxing for 30 to 60 seconds. Repeat the procedure. *Lower trunk and legs*—lift your legs 5 inches off the floor and tighten your stomach, buttocks, and all the muscles in your legs. Hold the tension for 5 seconds, then "Relax." Notice the relaxation spreading over your lower trunk and legs. Keep relaxing for 30 to 60 seconds. Repeat the procedure.

After you have practiced this routine several times in a relaxed environment, you will notice that it is easier and easier to become totally relaxed in shorter and shorter periods of time. When you are able to relax yourself in a reasonably short period of time (3 minutes or less), you are ready to begin using relaxation as a tool to combat periods of tension and stress. When you notice the tension and stress building, consider this a signal for you to focus on the feelings of tension in your body. Quickly tense your muscles, let them go, and then relax. Just like with all the other new habits you have learned, practice makes perfect!

Even if impulsive or emotional eating is not currently a problem for you, you should try this procedure for a while. It is not uncommon for people to deal very effectively with impulse eating during the program, only to notice that, after the end of the program, they begin to eat impulsively again and are unsure of how to deal with this. Such was the case with Hillary C., a 54-year-old real estate salesperson. After being on the program for 4 months, Hillary had lost 37 lbs and was very excited about losing the remaining 12 lbs and reaching her desirable level. She felt that her lowered weight made her much more effective in dealing with a wide variety of customers in the busy and often time-consuming business of selling homes. During Session 7, Hillary practiced the relaxation procedure on four or five occasions and felt that it would not contribute to her success. At the time, she was right. However, she noticed later that stress played an important role in her life when her daughter was about to deliver a baby. Hillary became very tense and anxious when she found that her daughter was in labor, and this state initiated an eating episode in which she, in fact, gorged herself. Initially, Hillary considered this to be a freak occurrence, but, approximately 1 week later, Hillary found herself eating potato salad directly from the refrigerator as soon as she walked in the door from a hectic day. Obviously, it was time for Hillary to review the stresses in her life and to deal with them more effectively. If she did not, it would seriously impair her further efforts to lose weight. Accordingly, she reviewed the relaxation procedure and practiced in the morning before work and several times during the day. Hillary found that, after 6 days of rather intensive practice, she could calm herself down relatively easily. The relaxation procedure served as an effective stopper of any future impulsive snacking. Other relaxation ideas that Hillary could have used include taking a hot bath and practicing slow, deep breathing.

Exercise

This week your exercise goal remains *1,500 calories*. Continue to record and graph the number of calories burned up during exercise, both daily and weekly.

Rewards

Continue to use the daily and weekly reward systems.

Homework

New Tasks This Week

1. Review together what happened at Session 8 as soon as possible after the session is over.
2. Read Handout 8 carefully.
3. Try the relaxation procedure several times next week.

Continued Tasks

1. Record all eating except free foods. At the end of each day, total and record your caloric intake.
2. Limit your eating to three meals (plus snack for child) each day.
3. Plan together your exercise for next week and record your plans on your Weekly Exercise Planning Worksheets. This week your exercise goal remains *1,500 calories*. Continue to record and graph your exercise as before.
4. Use stoppers or aversive imagery to limit extra snacks. Your goal remains no more than *two* extra snacks this week. Continue to record extra snacks as before.
5. Maintain good stimulus control: all food and eating only in the food areas; eating as a pure experience; a distinctive eating area.
6. Slow down eating and take a 2-minute time-out in the middle of each meal.
7. Continue your daily and weekly rewards.
8. Anticipate changes in your daily schedule and make plans to handle them.
9. Don't let others control your eating — be assertive!
10. Feel good about yourself and the progress you are making!

Chapter 10
Session 9.
Use of Goal Setting, Planning, and Problem Solving

REVIEW OF LAST WEEK'S WORK

Leader's Goal: To reinforce progress.

Activities: Small- and large-group discussions.

Discuss issues pertaining to stress presented last week, including trait thinking and the use of relaxation training.

SELF-MONITORING

Leader's Goal: To help maintain progress.

Activities: Instruction, discussion.

Review ideas about self-monitoring and graphing contained in Handout 9, emphasizing the importance of maintaining a permanent weight graph.

PROBLEM SOLVING

Leader's Goal: To teach systematic, flexible problem solving.

Activities: Instruction, modeling, practice.
1. Emphasize to the clients that they have now learned a new set of skills that they can always use in the future if they begin to gain weight again. If it becomes necessary, they can resume complete self-monitoring, begin a weekly reward system, and so on, until the problem is solved. The key point is that *they have the skills now; all they need to do is use them.*
2. Review the section on Problem Solving in Handout 9. If possible, see if someone in the group has a specific problem area you can use to illustrate the technique. If not, use the example in the lesson.

The five steps in the problem-solving model are:

(a) *General Orientation or "Set"*—recognize that a problem exists.

(b) *Problem Definition*—define the problem concretely in detail.

(c) *Generation of Alternatives*—brainstorm for ideas.

(d) *Decision Making.*

(e) *Verification*—try out the solution and see how well it works. Have a specific criterion for evaluating success or failure. If it fails, go back to step (b) or (c) as appropriate.

EXERCISE

Leader's Goal: To apply problem-solving techniques to exercising problems.

Activities: Brainstorming, discussion.

1. Set the minimum goal at *2,000* calories.
2. Spend some time dealing with what is going to happen to the clients' exercise programs when next winter comes. Use the problem-solving model to try to generate specific solutions for some of the clients.

HOMEWORK ASSIGNMENT

Leader's Goal: To get clients thinking about and working on relevant tasks during the week.

Activities: Provision of information and a handout, discussion of the week's work.

Continue to limit meal frequencies and helpings (one per meal); self-monitor food and exercise (2,000 calorie goal); use stimulus control, for example, by removing all food from the house except in the kitchen; use aversive imagery and stoppers to limit undesirable snacking; use chaining procedures (e.g., slow down eating); use positive pessimism; and practice assertive food refusal.

BEHAVIORAL CONTRACTS

Leader's Goal: To improve compliance.

Activities: Goal setting, discussion, writing of contracts.

Write a standard contract emphasizing any problem solving that needs to be done.

HANDOUT 9: GOALS, PLANS, AND PROBLEM SOLVING

This is the final handout of your weight-control program. In Handouts 1 through 8 you read about losing weight by modifying your eating behavior and increasing your energy expenditure. You also learned that by applying each of the steps described in these handouts, you can eliminate old, improper eating habits and learn new, more appropriate ones. You now have the tools that give you the ability to mold your eating and exercising.

In this final week, we will be concerned with the importance of continuing your weight graph — permanently — and dealing with problems that could arise in the future.

It is very important that you maintain your weight graph *permanently*, enter weights 1 or 2 times per week, and do not let the weight go up by more than 3 lbs, even after reaching your goal weight. While monitoring your weight, there are several important things to remember.

1. Keep your graph posted over your scale or in your closet with a pen or pencil attached. This will make recording an easy matter.
2. Try to weigh yourself at the same time each day. After you brush your teeth in the morning is a good time. Weighing yourself should become a biweekly routine. It is better to weigh with no clothes on. You could also wear a similar amount of clothing each time you weigh.
3. Women should be aware of their menstrual cycles and not be alarmed by temporary gains due to fluid retention.
4. Notice the trend of your recorded dots. Your daily weight will fluctuate (for some people as much as 3 to 4 lbs per day), but the trend is the important thing. It should be in a downward direction, staying close to your goal line.

Effective Problem Solving

Problems that are likely to develop in maintaining weight control vary considerably among different people. It is not feasible to anticipate all problems that could arise in the future and give a specific technique for coping with each problem. Also, these specific techniques might not work with other new problems that might arise. The following problem-solving strategy that is outlined is an effective procedure for recognizing, assessing, and coping with weight-control problems. Of course, like any skill, problem solving must be practiced carefully if it is to be effective. By learning this problem-solving strategy, you can gradually become your own counselor and solve most of your weight-control problems yourself. (This procedure can also be used for numerous other problem areas, for example, for problems between people.) Problem-solving skills should help you maintain over time the gains you have made so far in this weight-control program. This is very important because gains made in the formal weight-control program can be partially lost if you are not equipped to recognize and solve new problems when they arise.

Step 1. The Problem-Solving Model. The problem-solving model outlined next has five steps: (a) general orientation or "set," (b) problem definition and formulation, (c) generation of alternatives, (d) decision making, and (e) verification. These five steps are defined next, with examples related to weight-control problems.

1. *General Orientation or Set.* This means that you need to recognize that a problem exists and that you should try to cope with it. Problems are a normal aspect of living, but to deal with them effectively you can't act impulsively and you can't give up. When a new problem develops or an old problem flares up, you should actively cope with the situation in a systematic fashion. *Example*: "My weight loss has slowed down and I am getting discouraged. I can cope with this problem, but I need to carefully determine what is wrong and develop a specific solution for it."

2. *Problem Definition and Formulation.* This means that you need to define the problem concretely and classify relevant information, issues, and goals. This step is crucial and, indeed, there is an old saying that "defining the problem is half the solution." Your definitions should be concrete and specific, rather than abstract and general. Include plenty of details (events, situations, circumstances, feelings, and so on) in your definitions. Try to separate relevant from irrelevant details. Help from others is often useful during this step. *Example*: "Because my weight loss has slowed down, I must be eating more calories than I am burning up. Therefore, I need to reduce my calorie intake somehow or increase my exercising."

3. *Generation of Alternatives.* This means that you need to list the potential solutions or strategies for your problem. List several potential solutions before you try to evaluate or judge any of them (this is called *brainstorming*). Thinking of many alternatives increases the likelihood that you will come up with a good one. You might need to develop both specific and general solutions, but you will always need specific solutions for the problem at hand. *Example*: "I could cut out all desserts. I could start drinking my coffee black instead of with cream and sugar. I could increase my exercise level. I could try to switch to lower calorie meals."

4. *Decision Making.* This means that you need to pick the best solution or strategy described in the previous step. Try to anticipate the likely consequences of each of the alternative solutions you listed. Think of the personal and social consequences and the short- and long-term consequences. Sometimes the best solution is a combination of some of your alternatives, rather than a single alternative. Frequently, perfect solutions do not exist, and the best possible or lesser-of-evils solution should be adopted. *Example*: "I really like desserts occasionally and couldn't realistically stop eating them forever. Also, I am too

busy to increase my exercise level now. I think the best solution is to try to plan lower calorie meals and also to gradually reduce the amount of cream and sugar in my coffee over the next month until I can drink it black. To help do this, I will start self-monitoring my coffee drinking and start planning out menus for a week in advance."

5. *Verification.* This means that you need to try out the chosen strategy to see if it works. Give the solution a fair chance; try it several times. It could take practice and several trials for you to make the solution effective. Keep track (preferably in writing) of how well your solution worked. Have a concrete, specific definition of success, so that you can reliably tell how well your solution worked (defining the criterion for success in terms of something you can see and count is the best way to do this). If the solution you chose does not work, then recycle to Steps 2 or 3 and try, try again! *Example*: "I will try out this strategy for 1 month. If I lose at least 3 lbs over the next month, then my strategy worked. If not, I will go back to Steps 2 and 3 and try again."

We have included a Problem-Solving Worksheet at the end of the chapter. Use it to help organize your problem solving when coping with problems that may arise in the future.

Step 2. Exercise. This week your exercise goal is increased to *2,000 calories.* This 2,000-calorie level is sufficient to help maintain good cardiovascular function, and you should plan to stay at this exercise level *as a minimum* on a *permanent* basis. Maintain your weekly exercise graph on a permanent basis, to help you remain very aware of your exercising levels.

Step 3. Self-Monitoring. Until you have reached your final weight-loss goal and maintained it for *at least 3 months,* continue to record *what* and *how much* you eat in your Eating Diary, plus the total number of calories each day. *This is probably the most important thing you can do to continue to lose weight and reach your final weight-loss goal!*

Step 4. Slowing Down Eating. The 2-minute time-out in the middle of each meal is now optional. Continue to take small bites, put your utensils down while chewing, and concentrate on feelings of fullness during your meal.

Step 5. Rewards. Continue to use daily and weekly rewards to help you maintain your progress.

Maintenance Homework

1. Limit your eating to three meals (plus snack for child) each day.
2. Limit yourself to one helping of each food at each meal.
3. Record *what, when,* and *how much* you eat, including daily calories, until your weight-loss goals have been reached and your weight has remained stable for at least 3 months.

4. Exercise at a 2,000 calorie level each week and record it daily and weekly.
5. Continue to remove all food to the eating areas and to eat only in the eating areas.
6. Use stoppers or aversive imagery to limit extra snacking. Try to limit yourself to no more than two times each week. Record any extra snacks.
7. Continue to slow down your eating and concentrate on enjoying your food more. The 2-minute time-out in the middle of the meal is now optional.
8. Make your eating area more distinctive.
9. Use positive counterthoughts to counteract negative thoughts and excuses.
10. Maintain control over your eating—be assertive!
11. Remember that you now have the tools to lose weight and to keep excess weight off. If your weight starts going back up, reread portions of these handouts and start using the techniques that have helped you in the past. It is important to stay involved with your weight-loss group as long as you are still struggling with this difficult problem. The single most important thing you can do is to keep self-monitoring your weight and exercise levels. If you see a problem developing, use your problem-solving skills to find a solution as soon as possible. You can win the difficult battle to lose weight. But, you must be willing to keep working on it, permanently, in order to succeed—permanently!

FIGURE 10.1. Problem-Solving Worksheet

1.   *General Orientation or Set.* Recognize the existence of a problem. _____

_____

_____

2.   *Problem Definition and Formulation.* Define the problem concretely
and classify relevant information, issues, and goals._____

_____

_____

_____

_____

3.   *Generation of Alternatives.* List the potential solutions or strategies for
your problem. _____

_____

_____

_____

_____

4.   *Decision Making.* Choose the best solution or combination of solutions.

_____

_____

_____

_____

5.   *Verification.* Try out the chosen strategy and see if it works. Record the
results and any necessary modifications of the solution. _____

_____

_____

_____

_____

_____

Chapter 11

Sessions 10–100. Structures for Long-Term Group Treatment

As we emphasized in the introductory chapter of this book, one of the keys to successful treatment for weight control is the duration of the treatment. Relatively brief treatments produce limited and poorly maintained weight losses. We suggest maintaining your clients in weekly treatment sessions until they have reached their goal weights and maintained those weights for several months. For many clients, this will involve 1 year or more of treatment. The previous chapters provided structure for groups for 9 weeks. In this chapter, we will outline an approach that can be applied quite successfully for many additional months of treatment.

The basic structure used in the first 9 weeks of treatment can be utilized for all subsequent meetings. That structure includes three core elements:

1. *Subgroup review of last week's work;*
2. *Presentation of new information or large-group problem solving;*
3. *Formation of new contracts.*

The *review phase* works best by breaking the group into dyads or very small subgroups. This process is needed when the group includes more than three or four clients. It is crucial to make sure that each client gets adequate "air time." This facilitates appropriate maintenance of a therapeutic relationship, commitment to the group, and reinforcement of effort. In our experience, when there are more than three or four participants, these vital goals are not achieved without forming dyads (or triads) for the review portion of the session. It helps the dyads or triads if they are given an explicit focus for their discussions during the review phase. For example, you could ask each dyad to do the following: (a) identify specific problems each person encountered during the week (e.g., social pressures to eat, difficulties coping with eating in restaurants, lapses in self-monitoring); and (b) describe strategies and techniques that proved effective (e.g., imagery, assertiveness, stimulus control, planning). One member of each dyad could be asked to take notes during the review to add a touch of orderliness and formality to the process.

In the *new information or large-group phase*, the group leaders can work on some of the key issues and problems identified during the review phase. This often involves large-group problem solving (e.g., brainstorming, describing solutions that were effective for particular group members). The group leaders could also present new information during this phase about self-control strategies, nutrition, or exercise. In other words, this middle portion of the group allows it to remain dynamically responsive to new research findings and ideas. This strategy should help to keep the group interesting and appealing, rather than allow the program to stagnate, as do many nonprofessionally conducted weight-control groups.

In the final or *new contract* phase, each participant forms a new contract for the week. The new or noteworthy elements of each person's contract should be reviewed explicitly and publicly in the large group. This mechanism provides for individualized negotiated contracting and helps reinforce the learning that occurred during the session. It also helps maintain group cohesion and pressure.

This format can prove quite useful and flexible. Its usefulness is probably maximized if several group leaders meet regularly for peer supervision, supervision by an experienced practitioner, or just brainstorming. These meetings can add important concepts, techniques, and vitality to each leader's group.

References

Abraham, S., & Nordsieck, M. (1960). Relationship of excess weight in children and adults. *Public Health Reports, 25,* 263–273.

Beneke, W. M., & Paulsen, B. K. (1979). Long-term efficacy of a behavior modification weight loss program: A comparison of two follow-up maintenance strategies. *Behavior Therapy, 10,* 8–13.

Brody, J. (1981). *Jane Brody's nutrition book.* New York: Bantam.

Brook, C. G. D. (1972). Consequences of childhood obesity. *World Medical Journal, 3,* 45.

Brownell, K. D., & Kaye, F. S. (1982). A school-based behavior modification, nutrition, education, and physical activity program for obese children. *American Journal of Clinical Nutrition, 35,* 277–283.

Brownell, K. D., Kelman, J. H., & Stunkard, A. J. (1983). Treatment of obese children with and without their mothers: Changes in weight and blood pressure. *Pediatrics, 71,* 515–523.

Brownell, K. D., & Stunkard, A. J. (1980). Behavioral treatment for obese children and adolescents. In A. J. Stunkard (Ed.), *Obesity.* Philadelphia: W. B. Saunders.

Coates, T. J., Killen, J. D., & Slinkard, L. A. (1982). Parent participation in a treatment program for overweight adolescents. *International Journal of Eating Disorders, 1,* 37–48.

Coates, T. J., & Thoresen, C. E. (1978). Treating obesity in children and adolescents: A public health problem. *American Journal of Public Health, 68,* 143–151.

Coates, T. J., & Thoresen, C. E. (1981). Behavior and weight changes in three obese adolescents. *Behavior Therapy, 12,* 383–399.

Cohen, E. A., Gelfand, D. M., Dodd, D. K., Jensen, J., & Turner, C. (1980). Self-control practices associated with weight loss maintenance in children and adolescents. *Behavior Therapy, 11,* 26–37.

Collier, G., Hirsch, E., & Hamlin, P. H. (1972). The ecological determinants of reinforcement in the rat. *Physiology and Behavior, 9,* 705.

Craighead, L. W., Stunkard, A. J., & O'Brien, R. M. (1981). Behavior therapy and pharmacotherapy for obesity. *Archives of General Psychiatry, 38,* 763–768.

Dahlkoetter, J., Callahan, E. T., & Linton, J. (1979). Obesity and the unbalanced energy equation: Exercise versus eating habit change. *Journal of Consulting and Clinical Psychology, 47,* 898–905.

Dishman, R. K. (1986). Exercise adherence and dependence. In W. P. Morgan & S. E Goldston (Eds.), *Exercise and mental health.* New York: Hemisphere Publishing.

Donahoe, C. P., Jr., Lin, D. H., Kirschenbaum, D. S., & Keesey, R. E. (1984). Metabolic consequences of dieting and exercise in the treatment of obesity. *Journal of Consulting and Clinical Psychology, 52,* 827–836.

Dubbert, P. M., & Wilson, G. T. (1983). Failures in behavior therapy for obesity: Causes, correlates, and consequences. In E. B. Foa & P. M. G. Emmelkamp (Eds.), *Family in behavior therapy* (pp. 263–288). New York: John Wiley & Sons.

131

Edwards, K. A. (1978). An index for assessing weight change in children: Weight/height ratios. *Journal of Applied Behavior Analysis, 11*, 421–429.

Epstein, L. H., Masek, B. J., & Marshall, W. R. (1978). A nutritionally based school program for control of eating in obese children. *Behavior Therapy, 9*, 766–778.

Epstein, L. H., Wing. R. R., Koeske, R., Andrasik, F., & Ossip, D. J. (1981). Child and parent weight loss in family-based behavior-modification programs. *Journal of Consulting and Clinical Psychology, 49*, 674–685.

Epstein, L. H., Wing, R. R., Koeske, R., Ossip, D., & Beck, S. (1982). A comparison of life-style change and programmed aerobic exercise on weight and fitness changes in obese children. *Behavior Therapy, 13*, 651–665.

Epstein, L. H., Wing, R. R., Koeske, R., & Valoski, A. (1985). A comparison of life-style exercise, aerobic exercise, and calisthenics on weight loss in obese children. *Behavior Therapy, 16*, 345–356.

Epstein, L. H., Wing, R. R., Woodall, K., Penner, B. C., Kress, M. J., & Koeske, R. (1985). Effects of family-based behavioral treatment on obese 5-to-8-year-old children. *Behavior Therapy, 16*, 205–212.

Farina, A., Fisher, J. D., Getter, H., & Fischer, E. H. (1978). Some consequences of changing people's views regarding the nature of mental illness. *Journal of Abnormal Psychology, 57*, 272–279.

Felker, D. W. (1968). Relationship between the self-concept, body build, and perception of father's interest in sports in boys. *Research Quarterly, 39*, 513–517.

Flanery, R. C., & Kirschenbaum, D. S. (1986). Dispositional and situational correlates of long-term weight reduction in obese children. *Addictive Behaviors, 11*, 249–261.

Foch, T. T., & McClearn, G. E. (1980). Genetics, body weight, and obesity. In A. J. Stunkard (Ed.), *Obesity*. Philadelphia: W. B. Saunders.

Garn, S. M., & Clark, D. C. (1976). Trends in fatness and the origins of obesity. *Pediatrics, 57*, 443–456.

Garn, S. M., Cole, P. E., & Bailey, S. M. (1977). Effect of parental fatness levels on the fatness of biological and adoptive children. *Ecology of Food and Nutrition, 6*, 91–93.

Goldstein, A. P., & Myers, C. R.(1985). Relationship enhancement methods. In F. H. Kanfer & A. P. Goldstein (Eds.), *Helping people change: A textbook of methods*, (3rd ed.). Elmsford, NY: Pergamon Press.

Harmatz, M. G., & Lapuc, P. (1968). Behavior modification of overeating in a psychiatric population. *Journal of Consulting and Clinical Psychology, 32*, 583–587.

Humphrey, L. L. (in press). Family-wide distress in bulimia. In T. B. Baker & D. S. Cannon (Eds.), *Addictive behaviors: Psychological assessment and treatment*. New York: Praeger.

Israel, A. C., Stolmaker, L., & Andrian, C. A. G. (1985). The effects of training parents in general child management skills on a behavioral weight loss program for children. *Behavior Therapy, 16*, 169–180.

Israel, A. C., Stolmaker, L., Sharp, J. P., Silverman, W. K., & Simon, L. G. (1984). An evaluation of two methods of parent involvement in treating obese children. *Behavior Therapy, 15*, 266–272.

Johnson, W. G., & Stalonas, P. M., Jr. (1981). *Weight no longer: Keep pounds off forever*. Gretna, LA: Pelican.

Kingsley, R. G., & Shapiro, J. (1977). A comparison of three behavioral programs for the control of obesity in children. *Behavior Therapy, 8*, 30–36.

Kinter, M., Boss, P. G., & Johnson, N. (1981). The relationship between dysfunctional family environments and family members' food intake. *Journal of Marriage and the Family, 43*, 633–641.

Kirschenbaum, D. S. (1985). Proximity and specificity of planning: A position paper. *Cognitive Therapy and Research, 9*, 489–506.

Kirschenbaum, D. S. (1986). Obesity. In *Britannica international encyclopaedia*. Chicago: Britannica Centre.

Kirschenbaum, D. S., & Flanery, R. C. (1983). Behavioral contracting: Outcomes and elements. In M. Hersen, R. M. Eisler, & P. M. Miller (Eds.), *Progress in behavior modification: Vol. 5* (pp. 217–275). New York: Academic Press.

Kirschenbaum, D. S., & Flanery, R. C. (1984). Toward a psychology of behavioral contracting. *Clinical Psychology Review, 4,* 597–618.

Kirschenbaum, D. S., Harris, E. S., & Tomarken, A. J. (1984). Effects of parental involvement in behavioral weight loss therapy for preadolescents. *Behavior Therapy, 15,* 485–500.

Kirschenbaum, D. S., Stalonas, P. M., Jr., Zastowny, T. R., & Tomarken, A. J. (1985). Behavioral treatment of adult obesity: Attentional controls and a 2-year follow-up. *Behavior Research and Therapy, 23,* 675–682.

Kirschenbaum, D. S., & Tomarken, A. J. (1982). On facing the generalization problem: The study of self-regulatory failure. In P. C. Kendall (Ed.), *Advances in cognitive-behavioral research and therapy* (Vol. 1, pp. 121–200). New York: Academic.

Kirschenbaum, D. S., Tomarken, A. J., & Ordman, A. M. (1982). Specificity of planning and choice applied to adult self-control. *Journal of Personality and Social Psychology, 4,* 576–585.

Lauer, R. M., Conner, W. E., Leaverton, P. E., Reiter, M. A., & Clark, W. R. (1975). Coronary heart disease risk factors in school children. *Journal of Pediatrics 86,* 697–706.

LeBow, M. D. (1984). *Child obesity: A new frontier of behavior therapy.* New York: Springer.

Loro, A. D., Jr., Fisher, E. B., & Levenkron, J. C. (1979). Comparison of established and innovative weight-reduction treatment procedures. *Journal of Applied Behavior Analysis, 12,* 141–155.

Martin, J. E., Dubbert, P. M., Katell, A. D., Thompson, J. K., Raczynski, J. R., Lake, M., Smith, P. O., Webster, J. S., Sikora, T., & Cohen, R. E. (1984). Behavioral control of exercise in sedentary adults: Studies 1 through 6. *Journal of Consulting and Clinical Psychology, 52,* 795–811.

Mason, E. (1970). Obesity in pet dogs. *The Veterinary Record, 86,* 612–616.

Mendelson, B. K., & White, D. R. (1985). Development of self-body esteem in overweight youngsters. *Developmental Psychology, 21,* 90–96.

Perri, M. G., McAdoo, G., Spevak, P. A., & Newlin, D. B. (1984). Effect of a multicomponent maintenance program on long-term weight loss. *Journal of Consulting and Clinical Psychology, 32,* 480–481.

Perri, M. G., Shapiro, R. M., Ludwig, W. W., Twentyman, C. T., & McAdoo, W. G. (1984). Maintenance strategies for the treatment of obesity: An evaluation of relapse prevention training and post treatment contact by mail and telephone. *Journal of Consulting and Clinical Psychology, 52,* 404–413.

Phillips, D., Fischer, S. C., & Singh, R. (1977). A children's reinforcement survey schedule. *Journal of Behavior Therapy and Experimental Psychiatry, 8,* 131–134.

Polivy, J., Garner, D. M., & Garfinkel, P. E. (1985). Causes and consequences of the current preference for thin female physiques. In C. P. Herman, M. Zanna, & E. T. Higgins (Eds.), *Physical appearance, stigma, and social behavior.* Hillsdale, N.J.: Lawrence Erlbaum.

Sandifer, B. A., & Buchanan, W. L. (1983). Relationship between adherence and weight loss in a behavioral weight reduction program. *Behavior Therapy, 14,* 682–688.

Seltzer, C. C., & Mayer, J. (1965). A simple criterion of obesity. *Postgraduate Medicine, 38,* A-101–107.

Sjostrom, L. (1980). Fat cells and body weight. In A. J. Stunkard (Ed.), *Obesity.* Philadelphia: W. B. Saunders.

Stalonas, P. M., Johnson, W. G., & Christ, M. (1978). Behavior modification for obesity: The evaluation of exercise, contingency management and program adherence. *Journal of Consulting and Clinical Psychology, 45,* 463–469.

Stalonas, P. M., Jr., & Kirschenbaum, D. S. (1985). Behavioral treatment for obesity: Eating habits revisited. *Behavior Therapy, 16,* 1–14.

Stunkard, A. J., & Burt, V. (1967). Obesity and body image: II. Age of disturbances in the body image. *American Journal of Psychiatry, 123,* 1443–1447.

Thompson, J. K., Jarvie, G. J., Lahey, B. B., & Cureton, K. J. (1982). Exercise and obesity: Etiology, physiology, and intervention. *Psychological Bulletin, 91*, 55–79.

Wadden, T. A., Stunkard, A. J., & Brownell, K. D. (1983). Very low calorie diets: Their efficacy, safety, and future. *Annals of Internal Medicine, 99*, 675–684.

Wing, R. R., & Jeffery, R. J. (1979). Outpatient treatment of obesity: A comparison of methodology and results. *International Journal of Obesity, 3*, 261–279.

Wollersheim, J. P. (1970). The effectiveness of group therapy based upon learning principles in the treatment of overweight women. *Journal of Abnormal Psychology, 76*, 462–474.

Wooley, S. C., Wooley, O. W., & Dyrenforth, S. R. (1979). Theoretical, practical, and social issues in behavioral treatments of obesity. *Journal of Applied Behavior Analysis, 12*, 3–25.

Zinner, S. H., Levy, P. S., & Kass, E. H. (1971). Familial aggregation of blood pressure in children. *New England Journal of Medicine, 283*, 401–408.

Appendix A:
Application Form

PROGRAM OVERVIEW

Instructions: Make each of these points when first talking with both parents and children.

1. Research has shown that the components of this program are the most successful way to lose weight and maintain weight loss that has been devised to date.
2. This is a program in which the parent and the child work together, helping and encouraging each other.
3. The focus of the program is on actively learning new eating habits and changing the things in your home that help maintain bad eating habits.
4. There are *no forbidden foods* in this program, because it is *not* a diet program. We will, of course, be helping you to cut down on your eating and to eat a more balanced diet.
5. The program includes moderate exercises, which should be continued on a permanent basis along with the new eating habits we will be teaching. The choice of the exercise will be up to you, although we will encourage you to try to find some exercises or activities that the two of you can enjoy together.
6. A very important part of this program is the homework assignments you will be given each week. Some of these are keeping track of what, where, and how much you eat, recording and graphing your exercise on a daily and weekly basis, and keeping track of snacks.
7. During this intake procedure, you will both be asked quite a few questions. Please answer all questions honestly and carefully.

APPLICATION FORM

Parent's Personal Data

Name _____
     Last   First   MI

Address _____
          Street   City   Zip

Home Phone _____ Work Phone _____

Sex: Male _____ Female _____ Birth Date _____ Age _____

Marital Status: Single__ Married__ Divorced__ Separated__ Widowed __

Occupation _____

Educational Status (Circle highest year completed):

  Elementary School 1 2 3 4 5 6 7 8 9 10

    College 1 2 3 4   Graduate School or Professional Training 1 2 3 4 5

Height _____ Weight _____

How much would you like to weigh? _____

At what age was your overweight problem first noticeable? _____

How many times have you seriously attempted to lose weight? _____

Note below your degree of success with the three most recent attempts:

Approximate Dates
(e.g., Jan. 86–Mar. 86)   No. Weeks Dieting   Lbs Lost   Duration of Loss

Are you currently involved in any organized weight-control program? _____

  If so, describe: _____

Are you currently involved in any form of psychotherapy or counseling? _____

  If so, describe: _____

Are you currently making any active attempts to lose weight? _____

  If so, describe: _____

What do you think causes your weight problem?

_____

Below, please list the members of your immediate family, or others with whom you live, and indicate whether each has a weight problem:

Name	Relationship	Sex	Age	Weight Problem?

Indicate your response to the following questions by circling the appropriate number:

How much control do you feel *you* have in losing weight?

1	2	3	4	5	6	7
no control						total control

How committed are you to losing weight?

1	2	3	4	5	6	7
no commitment						total commitment

How ready are you to participate now in this weight-reduction program?

1	2	3	4	5	6	7
not ready						completely ready

Child's Personal Data

Name of child _____
            Last   First   MI

Does the child live with you full time? _____

If not, please describe custody arrangements:

Sex: Male _____ Female _____ Birth Date _____ Age _____

Current School Grade _____ Name of School _____

Current Height _____ Weight _____

How much would you like your child to weigh? _____

If your child is a girl, has she had her first menstrual period? _____

At what age was your child's overweight problem first noticeable? _____

How many times has your child attempted to lose weight? _____

Note below your child's degree of success with these earlier attempts:

Approximate Dates (e.g., Jan. 86–Mar. 86)	No. Weeks Dieting	Lbs Lost	Duration of Loss

Is your child currently involved in any organized weight-control program? ___

    If so, describe: _____

Is your child currently involved in any form of psychotherapy or counseling? ___

    If so, describe: _____

Is your child currently making any active attempts to lose weight? _____

    If so, describe: _____

What do you think causes your child's weight problem?_____

Does your child have any history (prior to 6 months ago) of emotional, behavioral, reading, or learning problems?

Yes _____   No _____

    If Yes, describe problem, setting, and duration of problem below:

Problem	Setting	Duration of Problem

Indicate your response to the following questions by circling the appropriate number:

How committed is your child to losing weight?

1	2	3	4	5	6	7
no commitment					total commitment	

How ready is your child to participate now in this weight-reduction program?

1	2	3	4	5	6	7
not ready					completely ready	

How important is it to you that your child lose weight?

1	2	3	4	5	6	7
not at all important					extremely important	

How motivated are you to help your child lose weight?

1	2	3	4	5	6	7
not at all motivated					extremely motivated	

How motivated is your child to help you lose weight?

1	2	3	4	5	6	7
not at all motivated					extremely motivated	

Parent's Medical Data

Check any of the following conditions that apply to you:

_____ diabetes _____ thyroid problem _____ colitis _____ ulcers

_____ hypoglycemia (low blood sugar) _____ hypertension

Describe any other conditions that would be (a) affected by dieting, (b) affected by exercise, or (c) related to weight control:

Do you currently have any medical problems? _____
If so, describe below:

Have you ever had any medical problems related to weight control? _____
If so, describe below:

Are you currently taking any medications? _____ If so, describe below:

(For women): Are you pregnant or are you planning to become pregnant during
the next year?

Child's Medical Data

Check any of the following conditions that apply to your child:

_____ diabetes   _____ thyroid problem   _____ colitis   _____ ulcers

_____ hypoglycemia (low blood sugar)   _____ hypertension

Describe any other conditions that would be (a) affected by dieting, (b) affected by exercise, or (c) related to weight control:

Does your child currently have any medical problems? _____ If so, describe below:

Has your child ever had any medical problems related to weight control? _____ If so, describe below:

Is your child currently taking any medications? _____ If so, describe below:

Mark with an X all of the 2-hour time slots during the week when you and your child *could* attend a group meeting.

	Monday	Tuesday	Wednesday	Thursday	Friday	Saturday
8						
9						
10						
11						
12						

	Monday	Tuesday	Wednesday	Thursday	Friday	Saturday
1						
2						
3						
4						
5						
6						
7						
8						

Additional Comments and Questions:

Parent's Signature

Today's Date

Appendix B:
Child's Interview

Instructions

This is an outline of a structured interview. The interviewer should complete each item as indicated.

Child's Name _____ Sex (M/F) _____ Age ____

Interviewer _____

1. After spending a few moments chatting with the child, see if she or he has any questions.

2. Do you think that you weigh too much? _____

   (If the child says no, ask why the child thinks she or he is here and then stop the interview. *This is sufficient to disqualify a potential client from the program.*)

3. How much weight would you like to lose? _____

4. Why do you want to lose weight? (Look for familial situations, social problems, physical limitations, etc.)

5. Why do you think you weigh too much?

6. Try to assess the child's motivation and the relative strength of the child's versus the parent's motivation. Is the child being pushed? In general, how enthusiastic is the child about this program?

(*Special Note:* Use the child's responses to questions 7–9 to screen for motivational, intellectual, reading, learning disability problems.)

Have the *child* read and answer the following three questions, including the Eating Summary (#9).

7. How important is it to you to lose weight?

   1   2   3   4   5   6   7
   not important   extremely important

8. How well do you think you will do in this program?

   1   2   3   4   5   6   7
   not at all well   extremely well

Comments:

9. What did you eat and drink today? In the space below, please write down *everything* you have had to eat and drink today.

Breakfast

Lunch

Snack

Dinner

Snack

Appendix C:
Parent's Interview

Date: _____

(Complete this as the *last* step in the intake process)

Parent's Name _____ Interviewer _____

1. Before interviewing the parent, examine his or her application form to see that all questions were answered and in sufficient detail. Look for odd or unclear items that need to be clarified.

2. Follow up on any items from the questionnaire that were unclear. In particular, pay close attention to the following:

    (a) Any medical problems the parent or child has;
    (b) Custody arrangements if the parent is divorced or separated, to make sure that parent and child live together full time;
    (c) Motivation of parent and child;
    (d) Child's past or present emotional and behavioral problems, if any;
    (e) Details and possible impact on our program of any other weight-control or therapy program parent or child is involved in. In general, if the parent or the child is involved in any other weight-control program, he or she will have to discontinue it to be in this program.

3. Follow up on any previous weight-loss attempts of both parent and child. Try to assess parent's attributions for success or failure and what he or she perceives to be the child's attributions for failure or success.

4. Try to assess the child's motivation. Make sure that parent is not coercing the child into the program.

5. Review financial arrangements with the parent.

Comments

Appendix D:
Sample Physician
Permission Form

Permission should be obtained for each participant prior to beginning work with that client.

_____ is planning to participate in a behavior therapy program for gradual and controlled weight reduction that is being offered by _____ . The program emphasizes change in eating behaviors and modification of the home eating environment and will include moderate caloric intake restrictions and increased exercise.

PHYSICIAN'S STATEMENT

I have examined _____ and have found him/her in sufficiently good health at this time to participate in such a program.

_____
Physician's Signature

_____
Date

Comments:

Author Index

Subject Index

About the Authors

Daniel S. Kirschenbaum received his PhD from the University of Cincinnati. He has published more than 70 articles based on his research and clinical work with a variety of self-regulatory problems, emphasizing obesity and sports psychology over the past decade. Dr. Kirschenbaum currently directs several treatment programs for obese people as part of his responsibilities as Associate Professor of Psychiatry and Behavioral Sciences, Northwestern University Medical School (Chicago).

William G. Johnson received his PhD from Catholic University. Dr. Johnson has been conducting clinical programs and research on obesity and eating behavior since the late 1960s. This work has been reported in more than 60 articles and in the series, *Advances in Eating Disorders,* which Dr. Johnson edits. Dr. Johnson is Professor of Psychiatry in the Department of Psychiatry (Division of Psychology) at the University of Mississippi Medical Center (Jackson).

Peter M. Stalonas, Jr. received his PhD from the University of Rochester. Dr. Stalonas died in 1985, after struggling during his entire adult life with the disabling chronic illness known as lupus. Despite his physical frailties, Dr. Stalonas managed to complete both master's and doctoral degrees in clinical psychology and to conduct a variety of studies, primarily on the behavioral treatment of obesity. This research resulted in more than a dozen publications, many of which are widely cited in the professional literature. Dr. Stalonas worked closely with both of the co-authors of this book on a number of research projects and publications. At the time of his death he was an Assistant Professor of Psychology at the University of Rochester (part-time) and a Research Associate at the University's Center for Community Study. The co-authors of this book, like all of Dr. Stalonas' friends and associates at the University of Rochester, were continually amazed at Dr. Stalonas' unyielding dedication to his work, his unselfish generosity and compassion, and his remarkable sense of humor and joie de vivre. He will be sorely missed. but never forgotten.

Psychology Practitioner Guidebooks

Editors

Arnold P. Goldstein, Syracuse University
Leonard Krasner, SUNY at Stony Brook
Sol L. Garfield, Washington University

Elsie M. Pinkston & Nathan L. Linsk—CARE OF THE ELDERLY:
A Family Approach

Donald Meichenbaum—STRESS INOCULATION TRAINING

Sebastiano Santostefano—COGNITIVE CONTROL THERAPY
WITH CHILDREN AND ADOLESCENTS

Lillie Weiss, Melanie Katzman & Sharlene Wolchik—TREATING
BULIMIA: A Psychoeducational Approach

Edward B. Blanchard & Frank Andrasik—MANAGEMENT OF
CHRONIC HEADACHES: A Psychological Approach

Raymond G. Romanczyk—CLINICAL UTILIZATION OF
MICROCOMPUTER TECHNOLOGY

Philip H. Bornstein & Marcy T. Bornstein—MARITAL THERAPY:
A Behavioral-Communications Approach

Michael T. Nietzel & Ronald C. Dillehay—PSYCHOLOGICAL
CONSULTATION IN THE COURTROOM

Elizabeth B. Yost, Larry E. Beutler, M. Anne Corbishley & James R.
Allender—GROUP COGNITIVE THERAPY: A Treatment
Approach for Depressed Older Adults

Lillie Weiss—DREAM ANALYSIS IN PSYCHOTHERAPY

Edward A. Kirby & Liam K. Grimley—UNDERSTANDING AND
TREATING ATTENTION DEFICIT DISORDER

Jon Eisenson—LANGUAGE AND SPEECH DISORDERS
IN CHILDREN

Eva L. Feindler & Randolph B. Ecton—ADOLESCENT ANGER
CONTROL: Cognitive-Behavioral Techniques

Michael C. Roberts—PEDIATRIC PSYCHOLOGY: Psychological
Interventions and Strategies for Pediatric Problems

Daniel S. Kirschenbaum, William G. Johnson & Peter M. Stalonas, Jr.—
TREATING CHILDHOOD AND ADOLESCENT OBESITY

W. Stewart Agras—EATING DISORDERS: Management of Obesity,
Bulimia and Anorexia Nervosa

Ian H. Gotlib—TREATMENT OF DEPRESSION: An Interpersonal
Systems Approach

Walter B. Pryzwansky & Robert N. Wendt—PSYCHOLOGY AS A
PROFESSION: Foundations of Practice

Cynthia D. Belar, William W. Deardorff & Karen E. Kelly—THE
PRACTICE OF CLINICAL HEALTH PSYCHOLOGY

Paul Karoly & Mark P. Jensen—MULTIMETHOD ASSESSMENT
OF CHRONIC PAIN

William L. Golden, E. Thomas Dowd & Fred Friedberg—
HYPNOTHERAPY: A Modern Approach

Patricia Lacks—BEHAVIORAL TREATMENT FOR PERSISTENT
INSOMNIA